Also by John Link

The Breast Cancer Survival Manual

Take Charge of Your Breast Cancer

Take Charge of Your

BREAST
CANCER

A Guide to Getting
the Best Possible Treatment

JOHN S. LINK, M.D.

An Owl Book

Henry Holt and Company • New York

Henry Holt and Company, LLC
Publishers since 1866
115 West 18th Street
New York, New York 10011

Henry Holt® is a registered trademark of
Henry Holt and Company, LLC.

Library of Congress Cataloging-in-Publication Data

Link, John S.
    Take charge of your breast cancer : a guide to
    getting the best possible treatment / John S. Link.
        p.   cm.
    Includes index.
    ISBN 0-8050-7056-7 (pbk.)
    1. Breast—Cancer—Popular works. I. Title.

RC280.B8 L533 2002   2002068541
616.99'449—dc21

Henry Holt books are available for special promotion
and premiums. For details contact: Director, Special Markets.

First Owl Books Edition 2002

Designed by Victoria Hartman

Printed in the United States of America
1   3   5   7   9   10   8   6   4   2

To the cure of breast cancer
and to all the women — past,
present, and future — who have
taken this unchosen journey

Contents

Foreword   xi

Acknowledgments   xv

Introduction   1

1 · You Are in Charge   7

2 · Demystifying the Disease   17

3 · Look before You Leap   30

4 · Treating the Whole Woman   46

5 · Your Doctor Is Human, Too   52

6 · Survival   59

7 · Saving Your Breast   68

8 · Weighing the Risk   78

9 · The New Era: Genetics and Breast Cancer   97

10 · The New Agents   105

11 · Never Again   113

12 · The Mind Is a Powerful Thing   118

13 · Faith, Healing, and Miracles   126

14 · Life with Breast Cancer   136

15 · Renewing Your Sexuality   150

16 · *Ikiru:* To Live   156

A Final Thought   161

References   163

Resources   169

Index   181

Foreword

Over twenty years ago I had the opportunity to meet Dr. John Link at a seminar he co-chaired entitled "Healing the Mind-Body Split." It was an exciting time in medicine because concepts of care and of the physician-patient relationship were changing dramatically. Norman Cousins's book *Anatomy of an Illness as Perceived by the Patient* had just been published. Patients were being encouraged to create a healing relationship with their physician by taking a more assertive role in the treatment process, and to actively evaluate the impact of the recommended treatment on their quality of life. Rather than representing a sabbatical from living, treatment was thus integrated into the context of the patient's life. These concepts formed a bridge between medicine and "healing," between science and technology and the unique individuals receiving these interventions. They placed the patient exactly where she should be, right in the middle of the fray. Her body is the battleground; the plan of attack is her own personal war. Along with these concepts, there emerged an enhanced understanding that treatment changes life forever. If the process of diagnosis and treatment guaranteed change, then the patient's ability to actively choose the manner in which her life was transformed was equally fundamental.

It was novel to hear anyone discuss medicine in this way, and I was particularly impressed to hear a physician speak of cancer in a manner that acknowledged and encouraged the full participation of his patients. My intuition that day about Dr. Link—that he is an oncologist whose perspective on the transformative power inherent in the crisis of cancer was formed by his experiences with his patients—has been abundantly confirmed over time.

Almost a decade later, I offered my services as a psychotherapist to Dr. Link to run the breast cancer support group. With each group meeting I had the opportunity to learn from wonderful teachers about what it means to live life informed by the profound awareness of its fragility. Amazingly, more often than not, I saw women emerge, phoenixlike, from the ashes of their trials, empowered by their experiences in treatment, clearer in their identification of what was important to them, and relentless in their pursuit of the people and life experiences that gave their lives joy. As an "outsider," I was awestruck by the laughter, sadness, longing, and passion that emerged as each woman found her own way through treatment and beyond.

In 1994, newly diagnosed with breast cancer and with an eight-month-old daughter, I had the opportunity to experience for myself both the terror and the blessings of this journey. I realized that for me to cope optimally with treatment, I would have to make the treatment truly my own. I researched and asked questions, built in safety nets and prayed. In this very individual process, each woman creates a path that is uniquely right for her. In Dr. Link I found a physician who not only supported my needs but also encouraged me to be an advocate for myself, to achieve peace through the process of diagnosis and treatment, and to live my life mindfully after treatment ended. Since then I have witnessed hundreds of women go through their own experience with breast cancer. Of one thing I am absolutely certain—that each patient defines for herself what she needs in order to make sense of, and to find meaning in, her experience. It has been a privilege to participate in the development of this book. My cherished hope is that it will prove a significant tool for women as they determine the role breast cancer will play in their lives.

Lisa Donley, M.A., M.F.T.

Acknowledgments

This book would not exist without the assistance of Lisa Donley and Kami Lakis. Both of these women have been instrumental in the entire process, from my original outline to the final draft. They have been my best critics and have given countless hours to the project. Both are breast cancer survivors and work with me at Breastlink. Lisa, a gifted psychotherapist, serves both our patients and our staff. By her example and teaching, she has made us better healers. Kami is the ultimate patient advocate. She is passionate, inspirational, and wise beyond her years. The book reflects their passion and dedication to helping women with breast cancer.

I am grateful to the entire staff at Breastlink for their compassionate care of women with this disease. Each individual in our organization contributes to our mission of delivering optimal, comprehensive care. I want to particularly recognize our CEO, David Delgado, whose integrity and leadership have greatly contributed to the success of the company. Susan Tanaka, R.N., Kami Lakis, and Lisa Kemp, R.N., do an incredible job as leaders of our three centers. I would especially like to thank each and every one of our nurses for her tireless dedication and compassion.

I am fortunate to work with brilliant physicians: Cynthia Forstoff and James Waisman, medical oncologists; Tomi Evans, Jane Kakkis, and Ken Deck, breast surgeons; Brooke Caldwell, Angie Sie, Nancy

Buccerelli, Chris Comstock, and Lauralyn Markle, breast radiologists; and Julio Ibarra and Lowell Rogers, pathologists.

I am extremely grateful to three men who have had a very positive influence on my life. My father, William Link; my track coach, Willie Wilson; and my medical school teacher Loren Stephens. All three died prematurely but left a legacy in their example and their teaching. To my mother, Jean, and sister Deb, your courage has been inspirational. To my sister Jennifer, thank you for being there with me. I am so grateful for the unexpected gift of our renewed sibling relationship. To my four daughters, Erin, Ashley, Amanda, and Brittany, the pleasure of watching you grow into beautiful young women only deepens my commitment to educating women and finding a cure so that you will never have to face this disease.

I would like to thank Mary Batten for her insightful review of the manuscript and for her encouragement. I am grateful to Sheree Bykofsy, my literary agent, and Deborah Brody, my editor at Henry Holt, for her assistance and confidence. There are many more people to pay tribute to, but most important, I want to thank those of you that I have had the privilege to care for through the years. Your courage and resilience are the substance of this book.

Take Charge of Your Breast Cancer

Introduction

As the medical director of a large, comprehensive breast cancer center in Long Beach, California, I developed a teaching manual for women newly diagnosed with breast cancer. This manual was originally handwritten, to educate women on the nature of breast cancer and the treatment options available. It was well received, and I was encouraged to formally publish the manual, which I did in 1998. *The Breast Cancer Survival Manual* is now in its third edition. I have spoken to and received thousands of letters from women who have been helped by reading the *The Breast Cancer Survival Manual*. But as good as that book is in helping women to understand and sort out their breast cancer, it does not convey the lessons in my heart and soul after twenty years of experience of caring for women with breast cancer. Some of the more vocal and feisty of the women in my practice have asked me to write a second book, one that would actually give women lessons in how to navigate their journey and allow me to speak from my heart about many unspoken issues that are critical to a full recovery and a better life. However, it was only after both my mother and sister developed cancer in the last eighteen months that I decided this new book needed to be written. I was, for the first time, on the receiving end of health care. I saw my loved ones being treated in managed care systems like commodities or liabilities, not as the incredibly valuable and unique individuals they are. I also wanted to relate some of what I've learned in twenty years of taking care of women with breast cancer that might be helpful to those presently beginning this unchosen journey.

This book is written for women with breast cancer—and for those that care about them. It will assist you in getting optimal care in a system where optimal care is not the norm. To achieve the best care, you must be educated beyond merely knowing about your cancer. You must also know how to approach your physician and treatment institutions to stimulate them to be their best, for your sake. This requires that you and your support network understand the medical system and the financial and political systems and values that impact what medicine defines as the standard of care. You want more than the "standard of care"; you want the best care. I have written this book to empower you to play as active a role in your care as you desire. I have to admit that I am biased. I believe that the more you choose to get involved, the greater a difference you can make in the quality of your treatment and, subsequently, the quality of your survival. In addition, when more women demand a higher standard of care, the bar will be raised and the care will be better for all women in the future.

Most women are terrified of getting breast cancer. It changes a woman's life irrevocably, and the treatment can be physically, emotionally, and sexually devastating. As you will see, though, this does not have to be the case. Society and the medical establishment often try to approach breast cancer as a single entity, and women are consequently treated as a disease rather than as the unique individuals they are. The good news is that 80 percent of women today are cured. Unfortunately, a significant percentage of women are overtreated and often return to their lives with permanent scars that interfere with their ability to live normal lives again. The sense of confidence and mastery with which a woman engages in the fight against breast cancer is, I believe, predictive of her ability to emerge from treatment not merely intact but enhanced by her experience.

All that you can ask for is to get optimal treatment at this point in time. What is optimal today may be replaced by a different and we hope better treatment in the future. We call this progress. Optimal care should be achievable regardless of the economic circumstances, the type of insurance, or lack of insurance one has. What is required to ensure your optimal care is that you must get involved. You must become educated and advocate for yourself. You can choose to have blind faith and turn over your care to the "system" and come out healed. However, I believe this is not a safe approach and you should not rely on it. In spite of "good doctors," and tremendous scientific progress, you should not blindly trust the system that is employed to take care of you. In the case of my mom and sister, I am convinced that neither one would have survived if they had done this. The truth is that you can make a major difference in the outcome, and the quality of your remaining life can be greatly affected by becoming involved.

The purpose of this book is to help you optimize your chances of dealing with imperfect systems and to give you the knowledge to make informed choices about your diagnosis and treatment. It is important to recognize when you feel unsettled or frightened and acknowledge how you feel. This will allow you to move toward action rather than being paralyzed by fear. There has been tremendous progress in the treatment of breast cancer, and that progress is ongoing. You want to be in a position to receive its benefits. No one will look out for you better than yourself.

You will define for yourself what is healing for you. For most women, the first step toward healing is medical treatment. The treatment process occurs at the most basic level, of human beings interacting in this crucible of illness we call breast cancer—the surgeons removing the tumor and repairing the defects, the oncologists administering new medicines and radiation to prevent recurrence, the psychotherapists exploring the psychological issues of stress and trauma. But there are larger forces that influence the treatment process that we have less control over but nevertheless must address. These forces involve the rapid development and emergence of new technology and how it is to be paid for. They involve the pharmaceutical industry, the health insurance industry, and the medical care delivery industry. Whether you belong to an HMO or PPO, your insurer does not have the right to dictate your treatment. Ultimately, healing occurs in the interaction between you and the individuals who care for you. A critical step is deciding, in collaboration with your treatment team, upon the *optimal* treatment for you. Once this is established, you can overcome the larger obstacles and impediments by advocating for yourself and getting those who care for you to do the same.

You certainly cannot trust the pharmaceutical industry, nor the insurance industry, nor the HMOs created to reduce costs. To some extent you *must* trust your doctors. They have taken the Hippocratic oath, which mandates that their sole goal must be to heal the patient. To ensure that optimal healing occurs, you must take charge of your breast cancer treatment. This book will help you accomplish this. It will suggest that breast cancer is not a single disease but is complex and requires analysis and treatment coordination among a number of physicians who should consider you and your cancer as unique. Treatment recommendations should be thoroughly explained to educate you about possible toxic effects, both acute and long-term, as well as potential benefits. In the end you will weigh the risks and benefits and come to the decision that is uniquely right for you.

The book will address issues of cancer cure: options regarding local control and assessment of the need for systemic treatment to prevent recurrence. It will address emotional and psychological issues that many breast cancer specialists refuse to consider, including treatment-induced hormonal changes and depression. It will also address issues of sexuality, fertility, and quality of life following a diagnosis and treatment for breast cancer.

I believe an important aspect of managing this crisis deals with control and trust. The only way to regain some control and be able to trust that the "right things" are being done is to take responsibility yourself. You will need to become educated to feel confident that you are receiving optimal care. Toward this end, I have taken the liberty of using examples from my own twenty-year experience as a breast cancer specialist. In all cases mentioned, I have been given permission from women, or their families, to tell their stories. Uniformly, these women are happy to share their experiences with others in the hope that it will be helpful. I have also used some personal experiences that have influenced me as a physician and healer. There is no substitute for experience. My hope is that I have been cognizant enough to sort out chance from cause and effect. We must be students of history—we must remember lessons passed down to us from our teachers and continually analyze our own personal experiences. Those that disregard history are doomed to repeat it. But more important, understanding historical perspectives and not regarding the past as dogma, but being able to build on it with new discoveries, is what makes progress.

One of my goals in writing this book is to help you establish and maintain healing relationships with your physicians. To this end, I discuss the coping mechanisms that allow physicians to care effectively for distressed and suffering patients over time without burning out. It is important to see your physicians as humans, with feelings and frustrations of their own, and as individuals who can learn from you. This relationship between the doctor and the patient goes both ways, and within the relationship there is the opportunity for growth and enrichment for both parties.

Some of the information in this book will become obsolete. The purpose is not to educate you regarding the latest treatment; it is to help you achieve optimal treatment, whatever it is at any given time. Our website, Breastlink.com, will be a good source for the latest treatment information that is not biased by the pharmaceutical industry or other enterprises that might have conflicting motives. *The Breast Cancer Survival Manual* is an information resource and is updated periodically.

As you read this book and go forward with your treatment and your life, try to keep things in perspective. It is important to address this experience with all the energy and resources you can muster. You are alive today and you will be tomorrow, so plan for it. Look at options in this regard, because, ultimately, decisions that are made will and can affect the rest of your life. In the heat of crisis, it is natural for you to feel the need to make a speedy decision regarding treatment, before you have sufficient data. Occasionally we see women make treatment decisions that are, from a scientific perspective, likely to place them at increased risk of recurrence. More often, we see women make decisions that lead to overtreatment or unnecessary treatment, the logic being that more aggressive and toxic must be better. You will learn that this is not necessarily true.

Although the pathway toward diagnosis and treatment of breast cancer is not anyone's choice, it is a major opportunity for emotional, psychological, and spiritual growth. As upsetting as this cancer diagnosis is, do not allow it to negatively dictate your life. You are in control and you have choices. There will be lessons to learn along the way that you can put to good use as you proceed. You may experience events and people much differently in the future. You will certainly make new friends. Keep an open mind to people and ideas. Let yourself love and be loved.

Once you have done what you can do, you can move forward with the confidence that you have done your best. Assume that you will live a full life, with the perspective of having survived a life-threatening illness. Pursue what is meaningful to you and embrace it fully. And last, though your situation is obviously serious, don't take yourself too seriously. Keeping a sense of humor is important. Face this crisis and all it involves with your arms wide open, your head held high against the wind, and laugh along the way.

You Are in Charge

> The idea of taking charge of one's medical program is the single most common practice among survivors. It is the cornerstone of a strategic recovery plan.
>
> —Greg Anderson, author of
> *Cancer: 50 Essential Things to Do*

This is a book for women with breast cancer. Its sole purpose is to help you navigate the medical system and receive *optimal care*. The dictionary defines *optimal* as "most desirable" or "favorable." I define optimal care as individualized or customized care that is neither undertreatment nor overtreatment for each woman's particular situation. It is a treatment that gives each woman the best chance of being cured with the fewest side effects and disruption to her life. I believe that as many as 40 percent of women in this country with newly diagnosed breast cancer do not receive optimal care. This is due either to misdiagnosis or to inappropriate treatment. Unfortunately, both lead to increased suffering and even, though rarely, death.

How can this happen? I don't believe it is intentional or done out of malice, but instead is due to ignorance, pride, lack of sufficient data, and miscommunication among doctors. In almost every case of mismanagement, a single physician makes recommendations in isolation or without accurate information regarding a woman's unique situation.

The recommendations often lack current scientific foundation and usually are financially favorable to the physician or the system under which he or she practices.

How difficult is it for a woman to receive optimal care in our present health care system? My experience as a breast cancer doctor seeing hundreds of women from across the country for second opinions each year is that a significant number of women do not receive optimal care. A significant percentage of women are over- or undertreated, with little consideration about who they are as emotional, spiritual, and sexual human beings.

· · ·

There is no question that your first priority is survival—optimizing your chances for a cure. Certainly, optimal treatment involves the best chance for cure. Treatment should be based on the nature of the breast cancer—its physical extent and its microscopic and genetic characteristics. With optimal treatment 80 percent of woman today should be cured, and this number is improving each year. These women need to go forth in their lives, feeling good and whole and able to live and love. Unfortunately, for many women, the treatment becomes worse than the disease. A confusing and unsettling paradox is that at the time the breast cancer is discovered, you usually feel normal and have no physical complaints. At the end of treatment, when the cancer is all gone and hoped never to return, many women feel sick and debilitated. Fortunately, their well-being returns once recovery from the side effects of treatment occurs, but some lose confidence in their body. Some women receive treatments that leave them physically, emotionally, and sexually scarred for the remainder of their lives. As you will see, this doesn't have to be the case.

To achieve optimal care, you need to be informed and become your own advocate. If you are the significant other of a woman with breast cancer, you can help your friend or loved one process information and advocate for her. Breast cancer is one of the few diseases that require a woman to make critical decisions about her own care. She can defer decision making or rely primarily on the advice of her doctors, but this unfortunately does not guarantee the best care.

Breast cancer requires the collaborative care of at least four or five different specialists, including oncologists, surgeons, pathologists, radiologists, radiation oncologists, and psychotherapists. Each of these professionals practices in the context of his or her own specialty and brings to the patient certain biases based on training, experience, ego, and monetary gain. For example, many surgeons believe that the more surgery, the better chance for a cure. This approach stems from the teachings of William Halsted, the father of breast cancer surgery. His operation, the Halsted radical mastectomy, was the only operation for breast cancer for sixty years. Although this operation is rarely performed today, the attitude that more is better persists among many surgeons. I've heard surgeons recommending breast conservation in public forums and in tumor boards (gatherings of various physicians and cancer specialists to discuss individual patient care), and then, behind closed doors, telling a woman, "If you were my wife, I would insist you have a mastectomy." The surgeon's training has focused on local control, and many were trained in an era prior to the use of systemic therapy—treatments such as chemotherapy or hormonal therapy—that impact the tumor cells regardless of whether they are confined to the breast or have migrated beyond the breast. Long-term survival of breast cancer depends on local control, but probably depends even more on controlling and eradicating the spread of the diseased cells.

I believe that the appropriate surgical intervention must take into account the risk of systemic spread and the necessity of systemic therapy. Surgeons often lose sight of the bigger picture, beyond the breast. This type of bias also exists in the other specialties. For example, in medical oncology, my own chosen field, it is common for oncologists to routinely prescribe chemotherapy to a majority of women with little chance of benefit. This advice, often presented as scientifically supported and necessary, frightens women who are in crisis. Many women don't even realize they have an option. When presented with the statistics of risk and benefit in terms they can understand, many women will decline the chemotherapy because the benefit is not worth the risk. Unfortunately many oncologists don't present women with options, but only with a recommendation. Many women conclude that if chemotherapy is recommended, it must be the standard and necessary. An emerging criticism of screening mammography is that the procedure leads to overtreatment of small cancers that are highly curable with limited surgery alone. Chemotherapists, like surgeons, get caught up in their own domain and forget to see the woman in her entirety.

Radiation oncologists also overprescribe treatment, particularly in older women. The standard is to give all women with breast cancer who have not had a mastectomy radiation for six to seven weeks. But this additional and potentially toxic treatment does not usually increase the cure rate. It does reduce the local recurrence rate, which is significant. Approximately 20 to 30 percent of women who do not receive radiation therapy will have local recurrences. If a local recurrence is discovered early, though, there is little risk of systemic spread. For women over sixty years of age, with completely excised tumors, the risk of local recurrence is approximately 5 percent.

Radiation therapy is usually presented as "absolutely necessary," and women assume it will increase their survival, which is usually not the case. Women need an honest presentation and then should actively participate in the decision to do radiation or not. If they passively accept the recommendation, they have missed an opportunity to decide what is appropriate for them. When a woman actively participates in a decision, I believe, she will feel less victimized by the treatment and will experience fewer side effects.

With this fragmentation of care, it is unusual for a woman to find a physician who will accept her as a partner and help coordinate her care, considering her as a human being who will be cured and go on with her life after breast cancer treatment. This is why it is important for you to be educated and to take responsibility for your treatment.

You may discover silent partners in your health care that you may not appreciate. These silent partners are the companies and financial interests that manage health care. With health care delivery constantly changing, people are now termed as "lives" that are bought and sold like commodities on the stock exchange. In many HMOs, there are incentives for health care providers not to treat. Doctors are *capitated,* which means they receive a small fee each month to take care of a person regardless of whether he or she needs or receives treatment. A certain amount of money is also set aside into what is called a risk pool, and at the end of the year, if this money is not used on tests or treatment, then the doctors will get a bonus. What is obvious is that the doctor gets paid more for not ordering tests or for doing less. Many of us went into medicine to care for people, but now it seems that some of my colleagues' major concerns are to avoid caring for patients. New terms such as "gatekeeper" have been added to our medical vocabulary. "Gatekeeper" is a terrible term. It refers to a doctor, usually the primary care physician (PCP) who controls whether a patient can "get through the gate" for appropriate treatment. The HMO system was initiated at a time when the cost of medical care was skyrocketing. It was seen as a method for cost containment by eliminating many of the excesses of medical care, including prolonged hospitalizations, expensive specialists, and the overprescribing of tests and drugs. In most instances HMOs were successful in keeping costs in line in the first three to five years of their existence, but costs began to rise again after this initial period. One of the problems is that the *Health Maintenance* part of HMO was not occurring. Patients' health problems were not being fully addressed, and diseases would resurface in a more advanced state. The cost to the patient and society was actually higher with the HMO system than the traditional "fee for service" system. I was aware of these problems from my patients, but I hadn't experienced this type of medicine firsthand until my mother became ill.

My mom, a vibrant, active woman, began to experience stomach pains and lose weight. She didn't want to bother me or my two sisters, so she scheduled an appointment with her PCP. She had seen her PCP on several previous occasions for routine checkups and liked him well enough. He seemed young and enthusiastic, and at the completion of their short interactions he gave her a nice hug, which she loved. She made an appointment regarding her stomach problem and was given a date four weeks later. The day before her appointment, she received a call that the doctor had a scheduling conflict and the appointment was delayed another two weeks. By this time, she had lost six more pounds, and she began to worry that something was really wrong. She finally got her appointment with her PCP, who was unconcerned. He ordered a blood test and prescribed a medication that blocked stomach acid production. Mom felt reassured, but worried in spite of her stomach pains actually lessening. However, she continued to lose weight.

When she dropped under one hundred pounds, she called me and confessed her plight. Hearing her symptoms, I feared that my seventy-four-year-old mom had cancer. I was on the phone immediately with her PCP, which initiated her referral to a gastroenterologist, who saw her within a week (without my intervention it would have been another four weeks). He put a scope down into her stomach and discovered an ulcerated large tumor. The stomach wall was markedly thickened. Using the gastroscope, he biopsied the thickened stomach wall as well as the edge of the ulcer. When she awoke from the light anesthesia, the gastroenterologist gave her a grave look and told her he thought she might have "a problem," but the biopsies would give the real answer. She would have to wait yet another week to receive the results, and she should schedule an appointment with her PCP.

My mom is a brave woman. She knew something was drastically wrong. She knew that she had a malignancy before the PCP told her it was true. The doctor was all business and had trouble looking her in the eye. He said the gastroenterologist's report, the CAT scan, and the pathologist's interpretation of the biopsy slides all confirmed she had a tumor. What made things even worse, he said, was that there appeared to be several spots on her liver that were consistent with spread to her liver. Later that night, my sister related the interview to me. As a general medical oncologist before subspecializing in breast cancer, I believed this to be a death sentence. My sister said the doctor tried to be positive and wanted Mom to see an oncologist to discuss possible treatment. "Is there treatment?" Mom had asked him. He assured her that there was tremendous progress in the treatment of all kinds of cancers. She asked him if he thought it would have made a difference if it had been found seven months prior, when she first complained to him of stomach pains and difficulty in swallowing. He said he didn't think so. She didn't believe him. He didn't give her his customary hug, but shook her hand and told her and my sister that he would be available.

Normally in an HMO, my mother would have had to wait several more weeks to see the oncologist, but her PCP pulled strings, perhaps because I was a physician, and Mom was able to see her within several days. Again my sister was with her. The oncologist was a middle-aged woman who was sympathetic but was obviously short on time. She apologized in advance for being the bearer of bad news. She told Mom she was terminal and that chemotherapy had limited value. In fact, she said, it would cause more harm than good. She made mention that she knew I was an oncologist and said that she was sure I would agree that chemotherapy was probably not indicated. She stated that she would be available to talk with me. She told my mom and sister that stomach cancer was incurable when it had spread to the liver. She further stated hospice was the most appropriate plan at this time, and my mom should get her affairs in order. The oncologist spoke in a monotone, without emotion, as if she were reading from a page in a book.

We came as a family to her, my two sisters and myself. What the oncologist had said, directly and without real compassion, unfortunately appeared to be correct. From my sister's account, I appreciated the oncologist's forthrightness and candor, nonempathic as it was. Many oncologists sugarcoat or misrepresent the truth, which can lead to toxic chemotherapy in the name of hope, with little if any chance of benefit.

In the next few days, my two sisters and I helped our mom sort out her things and get her legal documents in order. She divided the family pictures among the three of us. It was heart-wrenching.

I am relating this story for a number of reasons. In *The Breast Cancer Survival Manual* and in my practice I advocate that one should always consider a second opinion when dealing with information that is critical to survival. We were experiencing such grief with my mother's situation that we didn't initially think to follow my own advice. Although it seemed as if there was nothing to be done, I realized that we needed to be sure of the diagnosis, so I asked my colleagues in Los Angeles to review her slides and X rays.

I submitted the slides to my good friend Julio Ibarra, a superb pathologist whose specialty is breast pathology, and I took my mom's CAT scan to the radiologist at the hospital where I practice in Long Beach. The radiologist confirmed the large mass and tremendously thickened stomach wall, but thought the two spots on the liver probably represented cysts and not spread of the cancer. Shortly thereafter Dr. Ibarra called with incredible news. He had reviewed the slides and then had taken them to be reviewed by Jim Baker, a lymphoma pathologist, and they believed that my mom did not have a stomach cancer per se, but a lymphoma of the stomach, a rare malignancy that was treatable and perhaps even curable.

Once the correct diagnosis was confirmed, I was able to get my mom into treatment for her lymphoma under the care of my colleagues. This was not an easy task, but with my pressure on her insurance company, they allowed her to switch to an HMO that was associated with our hospital. Neither she nor I trusted her original doctors to treat her after they had misdiagnosed her.

Mom was under treatment for almost a full year. She had intense chemotherapy that caused hair loss, weakness, and mouth sores. This was followed by radiation that lasted five weeks. Her stomach tumor shrank immediately, and she gained weight in spite of the intense treatment. It has now been almost two years since her diagnosis, without evidence of recurrence.

There are some lessons here. *First,* although doctors may be competent and well-meaning, if they are acting on incorrect information, their treatment will be incorrect and the outcome will not be optimal. And once there is a critical mistake, interpretation of future information is prejudiced, based on the prime critical mistake. In my mom's situation, with the diagnosis of stomach cancer, the spots on her liver scan were assumed to be a spread of the cancer. However, once we realized that she had a lymphoma, it was unlikely the spots represented a spread because it is unusual for lymphoma to do this. Indeed, the spots represented two small cysts. *Second,* managed care may be good for containing national medical expenses, but it may not provide the best care for the individual patient. This type of system usually doesn't lend itself to collaboration and individualized care. Treatment is regimented and fairly rigid, based on guidelines. Roadblocks are placed to contain costs and reduce expensive procedures and treatments. A whole new layer of bueaucracy has been created to request and approve procedures and treatments in order to reduce costs. I believe that cost containment with HMO medicine may ultimately be a temporary phenomenon, with costs escalating later because of delayed diagnosis and treatment. The least of these costs is economic; the greatest cost is the unnecessary loss of life.

I honestly believe if I hadn't intervened in my mom's situation, she would not be here now. My actions did not require that I be a physician. Any well-meaning son or daughter could have gotten a second opinion. Since the initial diagnosis had seemed so logical to me as a doctor, I almost disregarded the advice I give to my patients to get second opinions and outside confirmation of a serious illness.

In my daily practice of breast oncology, I see on a frequent basis the same kind of mistakes from managed care: lack of communication and collaboration, denial of services, and plain apathy and burnout from individuals who once were idealistic and well-meaning. There are certainly good, competent doctors working in HMOs, but it is a system that frequently fails to care for the sick patient. This is not to say that all HMOs are bad and that the traditional "fee for service" system doesn't have its problems. The point is we have to pay attention to get the right care.

One of the things I do on a daily basis is to see women with newly diagnosed breast cancer for second opinions. We require a full review of all imaging (mammograms, ultrasounds, MRIs, etc.) and pathology. These are women and their families doing what we did for my mother. This requires being assertive and sometimes "pushing the system" or "ruffling feathers." Rendering second opinions puts me in a position to see the work and analysis of others, and I see mistakes. It is not my objective to create mistrust by writing this book, but to help women become more knowledgeable in their quest for the best care available. It is my great hope that women and their families will be aware of the appropriateness and necessity of advocating to achieve optimal care.

Be informed and aware. Be your own advocate. Demand the very best. *These* are the cornerstones of healing.

❧ 2 ❧

Demystifying the Disease

To understand where you've never been before, you have to
do what you've never done before.
—Kgmotsu Nkwe

The moment you learn you have breast cancer, your life changes forever. When you receive those most feared words, you enter an unchosen sisterhood. The very word *cancer* brings up images of suffering and
death. Fortunately, breast cancer does not equal death. Nevertheless,
in an instant, your wonderfully routine, mundane life turns into
chaos, and you know at some level that you're in trouble. The question is, how much trouble?

In order to be your own best advocate, you must understand what
you are up against. Education demystifies this disease, and greatly
helps in overcoming your fear of the unknown. The very process of
information-gathering is critical to your treatment, and at the same
time allows you to regain control. The fear begins to dissipate as you
begin to understand your cancer and how it is treated. You will begin
to feel safer as you realize that you have choices. Knowledge about
your disease is the first step to empowerment.

The first thing you need to learn is that breast cancer is not a
single disease. As much as the news media and even the scientific

community promote it as a single entity, it is not. You have to resist the temptation to believe everything you hear, because now that you have breast cancer, you will be barraged with information. It will come from every direction. From the newspaper and television: "New Break-through in Breast Cancer"; from well-meaning friends: "You must take this special herbal mix to strengthen your immune system." Everyone wants to help, but what you need most is accurate scientific informa-tion and a plan, based on your individual case, that will lead to cure.

The variations in breast cancer cover the spectrum. At one end, the disease can be purely noninvasive and 100 percent curable; at the other end, a highly malignant form will require aggressive, intense therapy, and the cancer can threaten your life. The treatment must be matched to the particular type of breast cancer that you have. Thus, there is potential for both overtreatment and undertreatment.

How Breast Cancer Begins

Your journey starts with understanding how breast cancer begins. Every new breast cancer starts with a mishap—a mutation in the DNA (deoxyribonucleic acid) of a glandular cell in the breast tissue. The DNA resides in the nucleus of each of your cells and is the blue-print for the production of proteins that determine the nature and behavior of that cell and every other cell in your body. It actually may take several mishaps to lead to the true cancerous transformation of the glandular cell. Some women have a genetic predisposition toward breast cancer, inherited from one of their parents. (This is discussed in more detail in chapter 7.) In a sense, each of their breast cells starts with the first mishap already in place. This is not the case for the majority of women, and we have little or no understanding how the DNA becomes altered or damaged in these nonhereditary, or what are called "sporadic," cases.

A breast cancer begins, then, in a single cell with a genetic mishap or a series of mishaps that create an altered cell that cannot complete its programmed life cycle, which includes cell death. Every cell in the body is programmed for a function and life span. Skin cells are produced from dividing cells at the basal layer and then work their way to the surface and are shed. Heart muscle cells never divide and last a whole lifetime unless they die during a heart attack due to lack of oxygen. A majority of cells, via an internal clock which resides in the DNA, at some point stop dividing and die a natural death, what we call *apoptosis*. The cancer cell is different. It keeps dividing and will not die naturally. But even worse, as it divides, it passes its altered DNA on to its progeny (future generations of cells). In the very near future, scientists will be able to analyze the genes of each cancer to determine the nature of the genetic mishap. This is called *genotypic analysis* of the cancer. Genotypic analysis is extremely exciting because it will represent the first step toward developing individualized gene therapy. With this genetic information, scientists will be able to repair an abnormal gene that is responsible for the cancer.

Genotypic abnormalities give rise to what we see under the microscope and how the cancer behaves. We call this the phenotypic nature of the cancer. *Phenotype* refers to the tangible properties, or physical characteristics, of an individual cell, group of cells, or even the entire organism that are dictated by the DNA blueprint. *Phenotype* is a word you will come across repeatedly as you read more scientific material about breast cancer. Today cancers are primarily categorized based on their phenotypic nature.

We have identified a number of phenotypic characteristics of breast cancer based on appearance, ability to spread, and protein receptors on the cancer cell surface. These characteristics have a relation to survival. Knowledge of these characteristics allows us, the medical establishment, to inform each woman regarding her prognosis, and it allows us to prescribe the most appropriate treatment.

As much as there is a tendency to lump breast cancer into a single entity, it is at least several hundred different diseases. Table 2.1 below lists the various phenotypic characteristics that allow us to classify a cancer for treatment decision making. I tend to liken this to "finger-

TABLE 2.1

Prognostic Factors

Age: <50 or >50	Cell Type: Lobular or Ductal	Grade: I, II, III	LVI: Yes or No	Node: 0, 1-3, 4+
Her-2: Low or High	DNA: Diploid or Aneuploid	P53: Pos. or Neg.	VEGF: Pos. or Neg.	S-Phase: High or Low
ER+: Yes or No	DCIS Present: Yes or No	BRCA1: Pos. or Neg.	BRCA2: Pos. or Neg.	EGFR: Pos. or Neg.
PR+: Yes or No	Marrow: Cells Pos. or Neg.	Size: T1, T2, T	Ki-67: Pos. or Neg.	Necrosis Yes or No

LVI: Lympho-vascular index: Special staining of the tumor to assess involvement of small vessels.

Her-2: Her-2 oncogene amplification of the cancer.

P53: Positive indicates a mutated gene and is associated with more aggressive cancers.

VEGF: Vascular endothelial growth factor production, associated with increased angiogenesis. (See also chapter 10.)

ER: Estrogen receptor.

DCIS: Ductal carcinoma in situ when extensive, associated with local recurrence after lumpectomy.

BRCA 1 and 2: Hereditary breast cancer genes 1 and 2.

EGFR: Epidermal growth factor receptor.

PR: Progesterone receptor.

printing" the cancer. There are at least twenty variables that impact the nature of a tumor and determine, individually and in relationship to one another, its aggressiveness. Some of the most significant are age of the woman, cell type, grade, lympho-vascular index, node involvement, Her-2/neu oncogene, DNA, P53 tumor suppressor gene, vascular endothelial growth factor, S-phase, estrogen and progesterone receptor status, in situ cancer, breast cancer genes (BRCA) 1 and 2, EGFR, bone marrow involvement, size of original tumor, Ki-67 status.

As an example of how we use variables, young premenopausal women tend to have somewhat more aggressive tumors than postmenopausal women. However, we see young women whose age variable would mediate toward an interpretation of a more aggressive cancer but have tumors with more passive qualities on other variables such as Her-2/neu or original tumor size. Some variables are more important than others, and new variables are under study. Cancer does not play by the rules—rarely is a tumor aggressive on every possible measure or more passive on all measures.

The heterogeneity of breast cancer may be appreciated when you calculate the number of different possible cancers created from the twenty variables listed in the table. The combinations total *1,769,472* possible different cancer situations.

Your breast cancer is unique to you. Many women, when they do visual imagery of their cancer cells, imagine these "super strong" cells capable of tremendous destruction. These cells can do obvious harm, but they usually are extremely fragile and will go into a "cell death" with minor injury.

In the early period of your diagnosis, when you are feeling most afraid and vulnerable, it is critical that you learn as much as you can about your individual cancer before launching into treatment. *The Breast Cancer Survival Manual* will be invaluable in this regard. The modern treatment of breast cancer requires accurate information about many aspects of the cancer.

My Sister's Story

‿ This lesson was reinforced for me when my younger sister, Deb, was diagnosed with breast cancer at age forty-nine. She has lived in New Zealand for the last thirty years, and in December 2000, she had a screening mammogram that was read as abnormal. She wasn't having any problem, but three weeks later, she was called back for further investigation, and at that time she was feeling swelling and fullness in her armpit. She was told she most likely had a small cancer in her breast, but it appeared to have already spread to her lymph nodes. The doctors performed a needle biopsy that confirmed she did have a high-grade cancer.

She called me immediately and had her needle biopsy slides, mammograms, and ultrasound sent to me by overnight mail. Meanwhile, in New Zealand, she was immediately scheduled to see a surgeon who wanted to perform a mastectomy and lymph node removal.

Her mammograms, ultrasound, and biopsy confirmed that she had an aggressive cancer that was dividing rapidly. Cells had already spread from the breast, and she had extensive involvement in the lymph nodes under her arm in spite of the fact that the tumor in her breast, at 1.8 centimeters, was relatively small. What I believed had occurred was that the cell or cells that had penetrated the lymph system and spread to her lymph nodes had further mutated and were dividing more rapidly than the original clone of cells in the breast.

My sister saw the surgeon, Dr. Caswell, who gravely informed her and her husband, Ron, that she needed extensive surgery and that it should be done immediately. They asked the doctor if he would be willing to speak to me, and he was kind enough to call me during their session. With my sister and her husband in front of him, he outlined his approach, which would be a radical mastectomy with a complete lymph node dissection because of the extensive lymph node involvement.

He stated she would certainly need radiation and aggressive chemo after the surgery.

Dr. Caswell was sympathetic and receptive to talking with me. I asked if he considered perhaps doing preoperative chemotherapy in order to shrink down the lymph nodes prior to an operation. This approach is becoming much more standard in the treatment of younger women with palpable breast cancer and involved lymph nodes. He said that his oncologists did not offer preoperative chemotherapy unless it was for inflammatory breast cancer, which my sister did not have. Inflammatory breast cancer is a rare type of breast cancer, usually seen in young women, that looks and behaves like a skin infection of the breast surface with swelling and redness and warmth, but it doesn't respond to antibiotics. The standard cancer surgical approach, a mastectomy, doesn't work and can be disastrous. If chemotherapy is given first, there is usually rapid regression of the cancer, and surgery becomes feasible. We learned this twenty years ago when we realized that chemotherapy given to rapidly growing cancers makes them shrink. I believed this is what my sister needed, but the New Zealand doctors weren't ready for this approach. Dr. Caswell went on to say that one of the newer class of chemotherapy drugs, known as taxanes, had not been approved for use in my sister's type of situation, even after surgery. He was almost apologetic, because he knew of the positive results that were being reported in clinical trials.

It was clear to me that breast cancer in New Zealand was treated with little individual tailoring based on a particular woman's situation. The socialized system in place in New Zealand was universally available, but it appeared to be run like a large managed care organization. New treatments were slow to be incorporated into standard care. My sister had had a previous encounter with New Zealand's socialized medical system when she developed multiple sclerosis several years earlier. Newer classes of drugs developed in Europe and North America were not available in New Zealand. One of these drugs, an interferon, had been of proven benefit in preventing flare-ups of the disease, and my sister had been active in lobbying the government to get it approved. The drug was approved thanks to her effort, along with those of several other advocates.

I was convinced after speaking with Dr. Caswell, and having reviewed my sister's imaging and pathology, that the best approach was chemotherapy prior to surgery. It was pretty clear that the New Zealand physicians were not comfortable taking this approach, and besides, they didn't have an important drug that would be helpful. Later that day, we decided to have Debbie come to our center in Long Beach for her treatment.

It has been an enlightening experience for me, as an oncologist, to have both my sister and my mother develop cancer. There is an unwritten law in medicine that a physician should refrain from treating family. With my sister and mother, however, I had no choice but to become involved. The problem with treating family is that emotional involvement can potentially interfere with objective decision making. Ironically, my patients and their loved ones frequently ask me, "If I were your sister or wife, what would you recommend?" I am always puzzled by this type of question because it seems to imply that many doctors would recommend a different treatment for their own family members. I was fortunate to have colleagues who were willing to take care of my mom and sister. I am grateful to them for their wonderful care.

My sister arrived to begin her treatment concerned that her cancer seemed to be rapidly growing. The lymph nodes under her arm were considerably larger than they had been three weeks earlier, when they were discovered. I consoled her that this might work to our advantage, in that fast-growing cancers were highly sensitive to chemotherapy. Debbie was also concerned that mammography had not discovered her cancer in an early state.

I explained to her that screening mammography is not a perfect test. Approximately 10 percent of breast cancers will not show up on a mammogram even when they are palpable. Some fast-growing cancers become palpable before a woman is due for her next mammo-gram. These are called *interval cancers*. In her case, even though the cancer was nonpalpable in the breast, it had spread to the lymph nodes, and they rapidly became palpable. This is quite unusual and reflects the aggressiveness of her malignancy.

Due to the aggressiveness of her tumor, it was clear that she would need systemic therapy with chemotherapy. Systemic treatment involves giving medicines such as chemotherapy, antibody therapy, and/or hor-monal therapy to the patient, either by pill or intravenously. These medicines are then disseminated through the body via the blood cir-culatory system. We call this *adjuvant* systemic therapy when it is given after surgery.

I explained to my sister that the time to treat a tumor is when the number of cells that have escaped is at a minimum. The primary goal is to kill any cells that may have escaped into the system. In her case we felt that chemotherapy needed to be started before surgery (*neo-adjuvant* chemotherapy). We would have proof that the drugs were working by observing the response of the lymph nodes. When cells leave the primary breast cancer and penetrate a blood vessel, they most often end up in areas of the body that have large amounts of small blood vessels, such as the lung, the liver, and the bone marrow.

The pathology report from your breast biopsy contains the critical information that allows your physicians to analyze your situation and develop an optimal treatment plan. In your mother's generation, there was only one treatment for all breast cancer, and that was a mastectomy. It didn't matter that there were different kinds of breast cancer, because there was only one treatment. Fortunately, we have a number of types of treatments and many more on the way. Optimal treatment depends on understanding the heterogeneity of breast can-cer. The critical information necessary for treatment planning can often be obtained from imaging studies and needle biopsies. Table 2.2 (page 26) lists what I consider the important characteristics of a breast cancer that aid in treatment planning.

TABLE 2.2

Breast Cancer Characteristics
for Treatment Planning

Size of Invasive Tumor	The size of the tumor is critical for determining if breast conservation is feasible. Size is also a predictor of spread to lymph and blood.
Lymph Node Status	The involvement of the draining regional lymph nodes by cancer is the most powerful predictor we have for systemic involvement. Almost all women with nodal involvement will be recommended for some type of systemic therapy.
Histologic Grade	Histologic grade is a predictor of the aggressiveness of a cancer. It correlates to responsiveness to chemotherapy. The higher the grade, the more responsive to chemo.
Her-2 Oncogene	When Her-2 oncogene is overproduced, the cancer is more aggressive. Treatment with a new antibody drug known as Herceptin is called for.
Hormone Receptors	Breast cancer cells may have receptors on their cell surfaces for the hormones estrogen and progesterone. The presence of these receptors predicts that hormonal treatment interventions can prevent recurrence.

The Malignant Cell

◌ All breast cancers originate in the glandular cells that form either the milk ducts or the terminal lobular buds that produce milk under hormonal influence (see figure 2.1). The mutated breast glandular cell that becomes a cancer can retain some of the characteristics of the original healthy glandular cell, including hormone receptors for estrogen or progesterone on the cell surface. I believe that if the cancer retains these estrogen receptors, it can be stimulated or inhibited by manipulating the hormonal environment. Thus, knowing the tumor's hormone receptor status is a critical factor in treatment planning. If

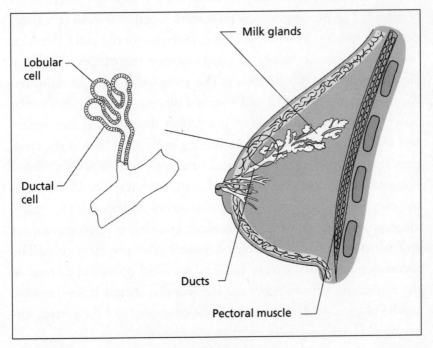

FIGURE 2.1
Breast ducts and lobular cells

the cancer cell looks microscopically similar to the cell of its origin, it is termed well differentiated, and it usually retains some normal functions that involve proteins like hormone receptors. If the cancer cell is microscopically more dissimilar or undifferentiated from the normal breast cell, it may not express many of the normal proteins. In fact, it may produce excess amounts of certain proteins that stimulate accelerated growth, angiogenesis (the production of blood vessels), and cell division. As we learn more about these proteins and growth factors, we will be able to produce drugs that can counteract them and will prevent recurrence. In chapter 10, you will learn the amazing story of Herceptin, a new drug that acts against a specific overproduced growth factor in some types of breast cancer.

Breast cancer treatment now requires much more than a knowledge of surgical technique. It requires a knowledge of the heterogeneity of breast cancer, including its biochemistry, genetics, and patterns of spread. The treating doctors must work together to deliver optimal care. The surgeon must rely on the mammographer to make the diagnosis with a needle biopsy and then localize the cancer to achieve clear margins around the tumor. The pathologist must confirm that the margins are clear, to avoid a second surgery. The surgeon must be concerned about the spread of the cancer through the duct system and attempt to remove the surrounding milk ducts, but at the same time leave a good cosmetic result. I frequently see women for second opinions whose operating surgeons have not even reviewed the mammogram prior to surgery. Even worse, surgeons will operate on a mammographic or palpable breast lesion not knowing yet that it is cancer and actually cut into the tumor, potentially spreading cells. The incompletely excised cancer requires a second operation to remove the remaining portion and clear the margins. A much less invasive needle biopsy could have provided the diagnosis, and the correct surgery could have been performed on the first try.

As in my sister's situation, it may be safer to treat the cancer with systemic therapy prior to doing the definitive surgery for local control.

There are both theoretic and real advantages in this approach for women with larger aggressive tumors.

· · ·

The diagnosis and treatment of breast cancer has become much more complex than it was a few years ago. Centers of excellence have emerged where specialists from different disciplines work together to achieve optimal results and include you, the patient, in the treatment decision process. It is important that you are not assigned the disease of breast cancer without consideration of your unique situation. With the crisis of the diagnosis, there is usually a sense of panic and urgency to begin treatment. Before you begin this journey, however, you may want to take a little extra time and make sure your team is collaborating and there is a plan.

∞ 3 ∞

Look before You Leap

Even if you're on the right track, you'll get run over if you just stand there.

—Will Rogers

With a breast cancer diagnosis, your world is suddenly turned upside down. For most women there is a burning desire for someone to tell them everything will be okay. Your short-term fear says, "Just help me to feel safe." Your long-term best interest lies in methodically pursuing the best available data about your cancer and its treatment. Ultimately, safety comes from the knowledge that you have pursued the best treatment available for your type of breast cancer. To achieve this result, you shouldn't blindly launch into treatment without having your case reviewed by a physician or group of physicians who specialize in breast cancer treatment. It is important to look before you leap. With major advances in technology, many of the standard treatments for breast cancer are being replaced by newer, more effective approaches. You want to feel confident that the treatment that is recommended is right for your individual situation.

How do you know you are getting the right treatment? Knowing your own disease is not enough. You must understand the forces that stimulate physicians to provide an optimal level of performance, which you must demand. But first you must know what to demand. This chapter will discuss the forces that influence medicine. You will come to know how you, the individual patient, are impacted by the system. In doing so, you will begin to know what to demand and how to demand it.

The Importance of a Second Opinion

꩜ The best assurance that the right treatment is being advised is to get a second opinion from a multidisciplinary breast cancer team. You must take the time, extend the effort, and incur the expense, if you want it to be productive. Your goal is to confirm that the information about your cancer is accurate, that all appropriate interventions have been considered, and that the proposed treatment plan is optimal for your individual situation.

You don't want to be recruited into an institution's special research protocol unless you're convinced it's the most appropriate treatment for you. Nor do you want to be told what a physician thinks you want to hear in order to attract you to his or her treatment facility. You need an independent, objective review of your case, rendered by a team that will not actually be administering the treatment. As alluded to in the previous chapter, if you were this doctor's loved one, what would he or she recommend as optimal treatment? I am not suggesting that the doctors who diagnosed the cancer and are making treatment recommendations are wrong or will mistreat you. On the contrary, in most cases the original doctors have made the correct diagnosis and offered the best treatment plan. Most women will return to their "home team," so to speak, after they have confirmation that they are on the right path. It is not unusual for the consulting team to make some minor revisions in pathologic interpretation or treatment. This should not be considered a reason for loss of confidence in your original team.

Breast cancer management requires at least six different specialists—surgeon, radiologist, pathologist, radiation and medical oncologists, plastic surgeon—working together. Most problems begin when there is little communication among these specialists.

I frequently see this lack of collaboration when I consult on a second opinion. Recently our team saw Jill, a young woman with a family history of breast cancer, who had a fairly extensive abnormal area in her right breast. She underwent a biopsy, at an outside facility, that was interpreted by the pathologist as low grade in situ, preinvasive breast cancer. We reviewed her outside biopsy slides, her mammograms, and did a complete history and exam. Our pathologist interpreted the slides as showing ductal hyperplasia with atypia. This means that the breast ductal cells were abnormal with precancerous changes, but were not in fact cancer, as the outside pathologist had reported. Since this is a difficult area of breast pathology, we were not particularly critical of the outside pathologist for his incorrect assessment.

Jill's mother had had a breast cancer at age forty-six, and her mother's only sister had had both breast cancer and ovarian cancer. The two sisters' mother died of a stroke at age eighty-seven. However, their father's sister had a breast cancer at forty-three and died of metastatic breast cancer at fifty-one. We suspected, given Jill's family history, that she might have one of the hereditary breast cancer genes, either BRCA 1 or 2. The atypical ductal hyperplasia (ADH), although not cancer, does increase her subsequent risk of breast cancer (see also chapter 9). Based on her age, the biopsy, and her family history, we recommended she have genetic testing. This was performed and three weeks later the result returned revealing she was positive for the BRCA1 gene. With the ADH and the positive gene we estimated her risk of breast cancer at approximately 80 to 90 percent over the next ten years.

After having our team review all the data, I sat down with Jill and her husband and we discussed the results of her testing and the options for management that we might consider. What initially seemed to be a problem of a preinvasive breast cancer turned out not to be cancer.

Our team approach allowed us to give her the correct diagnosis and discover that she had inherited a gene that substantially increased her risk of breast cancer. With this information she had two options available to her. She could have bilateral mastectomies, which would remove almost all of her breast tissue prior to a cancer developing, thus greatly reducing her risk. Studies suggest that with this treatment her breast cancer risk would be reduced from 80 percent to less than 5 percent. The other option would be to proceed with vigilant breast cancer surveillance, through mammography, ultrasound, and perhaps MRI testing. This would not reduce her risk but would allow for early detection of a breast cancer.

Presently, Jill is studying her options. She has seen several plastic surgeons and has interviewed a young woman who underwent breast removal with immediate reconstruction.

Multidisciplinary Review

The ideal situation occurs when your doctors can sit down together and review your case, including your family history, look at your mammograms and biopsy, and discuss the best approach. We call this the "pretreatment planning conference" or multidisciplinary review. This type of care takes time and commitment on your part and on the part of your physicians. If a treating physician works in a vacuum without reviewing the material and without having input from colleagues, mismanagement is more likely to occur.

You need someone who can see the big picture. Optimal care requires that the physician not be inhibited by what I call "specialty blinders." To quote the famous psychologist Abraham Maslow, "If the only tool you have is a hammer, you tend to see every problem as a nail." This attitude is unfortunately all too commonplace among specialists. They want to help and want to do good, but are trained to do only one thing well. This predicament was once thought to be primarily a problem of surgeons, but it also occurs among radiation and medical oncologists, as well as plastic surgeons.

Another inhibitor to receiving optimal care is that many physicians don't know about the changes that are occurring in breast cancer treatment. As medicine evolves rapidly, new and innovative treatments become the standard, and ineffective, older treatments are discarded. You want your physicians to be experienced, but also willing to keep up with progress. As the patient, you won't want to be the first on which the new is tried or the last before the old is put aside. The greater a doctor's experience, the more objective he or she can be regarding the effectiveness of a new treatment. We doctors tend to be creatures of habit, but evolution requires innovation. Table 3.1 shows areas of emerging technology in breast cancer care. Some are very new and are undergoing evaluation in clinical trials to determine their worth. Others are further along and are rapidly becoming standard.

TABLE 3.1

New Innovations in Breast Cancer

Area	Innovation	Description
Prevention	SERMs (Selective Estrogen Receptor Modulator)	This class of drug interferes with estrogen stimulation of breast glandular cells and probably reverses pre-malignant changes in hormone sensitive cells. We now know that SERMs prevent certain types of breast cancer. With this knowledge, pharmaceutical companies are developing the perfect HRT in a SERM that will have all of the positive effects of estrogen on the bones and heart, without increasing cancer risk.
	Vaccines	These agents stimulate the immune recognition of malignant cells and allow for targeted cell deaths. Though none of these agents is FDA-approved yet, there are numerous clinical trials in progress.

Area	Innovation	Description
Screening and Imaging	Digital Mammography	Available but expensive. Digital has advantages over regular mammography for storage and reconfiguring images. No increased detection rate so far.
	Computerized Mammographic Interpretation	Provides a second computer reading of the mammogram along with the radiologist's interpretation. Studies indicate an increase in cancer detection rate.
	Positive Emission Tomography (PET Scanning)	A dynamic imaging technique using a radioactive tracer tagged to a unique sugar that is taken up by cancer cells. Approved by Medicare in 2002 to find and follow systemic spread.
Surgery	Magnetic Resonance Imaging (MRI)	Special MRI technology has been developed to image breasts and has shown very promising results in high-risk women with dense breasts. It is also useful in assessing the extent of cancer prior to surgery for proper treatment planning.
	Sentinel Lymph Node Staging	This procedure uses blue dye and radioactive tracers to identify the first draining lymph node. It is rapidly becoming the standard of care for staging of lymph node involvement in early breast cancer. Prevents excessive surgery that can cause swelling of the arm (lymphedema).
	Bone Marrow Staging	Bone marrow is analyzed to isolate cancer cells. Studies suggest this very sensitive test predicts early systemic involvement. The technology may replace lymph node staging as the key indicator of cure.
	Skin Sparing Mastectomy	Removal of breast glandular tissue without removing skin. The technique allows for a superior cosmetic result with fewer visible scars and a more natural-appearing reconstructed breast.

Area	Innovation	Description
Surgery	Free Tissue Transfer	Surgical technique of transferring fat from abdomen or buttocks to form a breast. Uses special micro-surgical technique to reconnect blood vessels. It is a reconstructive option using natural tissue instead of synthetic material. Another benefit is that this single surgery usually prevents future complications seen with implant surgery.
Radiation	Irridium Afterloading	Radioactive seeds are inserted through a catheter into the tumor cavity after the cancer is removed. Pilot studies show that for unifocal, ductal cancers, the efficacy of this treament, which lasts for 5 days, is equal to the 6 to 7 weeks of conventional external beam radiation. The seeds are inserted daily for a short period of time and are then removed. This is all done in an outpatient setting.
Therapeutics	Hormonal Intervention	There have been many recent developments in the treatment of hormone receptor–positive cancer. Faslodex blocks the hormone receptor development process, which starves the tumor cell of the hormone and leads to cell death. A new class, the aromatase inhibitors, blocks the key enzyme in cells responsible for estrogen production, resulting in cell death through estrogen deprivation.
	Chemo-therapy	There is continuing progress in reducing the toxicity of chemotherapy and determining combinations of drugs that have synergy, i.e., they do more together than as single agents. Docotaxel (Taxotere) and capecitabine (Xeloda) are being added to standard regimens. Biologics such as Iterceptin are being combined with chemotherapy.
	Biologics and Gene Therapies	The major area of research today. Natural "growth factors" that stimulate tissue healing, including the immune system and the bone marrow, to aid in repair from treatment. On the cancer treatment side, antibodies such as Herceptin and RhuVEGF block growth and prevent angiogenesis.

Your treating or consulting oncologist should keep you aware of new treatments that might improve your outcome. This may involve participation in a clinical trial. With information and education you can make an "informed consent" regarding any new treatment for which you may be eligible.

How to Get the Most Current Treatment

⊙ Up till now in this chapter, I have been addressing how you, the individual, can get the best care. The next question you must answer is: "How do I ensure that my physicians continue to acquire and maintain knowledge of and deliver the state of the art in medicine as it applies to my care?" In asking this question, you should be aware that even in medical science there are forces that resist progress and change. Some of these forces are financial, because the new is usually expensive. When a pharmaceutical company introduces a drug, it has exclusive rights to produce the drug for a number of years (usually five to seven), and the price it charges is high. Some of the high cost is justified, as the company must recoup the research and development cost of bringing the drug to the marketplace, which involves proving that the drug or device enhances the treatment of a disease. A number of rigorous trials must be conducted. In oncology this involves comparing a new medicine or treatment with an existing standard treatment.

Physicians often resist trying new treatments or procedures. This is particularly true if it is a procedure that requires retraining. There is comfort in sticking with the familiar, since change requires energy, time, and often risk. An example is the use of "sentinel lymph node staging" to stage early breast cancer. This new technique identifies the first draining node, the *sentinel node*, of the cancer and requires the use of a small amount of radioactive material along with a blue dye injected adjacent to the cancer. Both the dye and the radioactive tracer flow to the sentinel node in the same manner that fluid from the breast flows to this node. The sentinel node is the initial site to which cancer cells will spread from the breast. When the two agents hit the sentinel node, it becomes a blue color and emits a signal that can be detected by a radioactive sensor. The node is then removed for pathologic analysis, which will reveal whether or not there is cancer present. The radioactive material safely dissipates from the body after the sentinel node has been identified. When this node is free of cancer, the rest of the nodes will likely show no cancer involvement. The patient will benefit if the sentinel node is negative, because the surgeon can avoid removing multiple nodes, which can lead to significant side effects such as pain, nerve damage, and chronic swelling. Surgeons trained to do the traditional full lymph node removal have been slow to use this technological advance. Be sure to ask your oncologist about the method of lymph node sampling that the surgeon will use in your case. There is a learning curve in performing this procedure, which usually involves performing ten to twenty sentinel lymph node dissections under the mentoring of a surgeon who is experienced in this technique.

It took approximately five years for the sentinel lymph node technique to go from a research protocol to a widely accepted standard procedure. New drugs reach the oncologist's practice even more rapidly, because pharmaceutical companies are extremely aggressive in marketing these drugs to doctors. The major companies have marketing divisions with large numbers of sales representatives who call on the physicians' offices to promote drugs their company produces. These "reps," usually attractive, knowledgeable, and friendly, provide literature and samples to familiarize the physician and the office staff with a particular new drug or treatment. Many pharmaceutical companies will offer a potential prescribing physician a trip to a resort for an educational seminar on the new treatment. During these seminars the company has a captive audience to market its product. There are fancy dinners and rounds of golf and often a stipend given to the physicians for their time. The industry spends many thousands of dollars a year per physician to promote its products. Though this is a seductive approach, it is not the optimal way for physicians to learn about a new drug or treatment.

You want to be treated by a team of physicians who gain their knowledge by attending the appropriate national and international conferences, reading peer-reviewed scientific journals, and practicing up-to-date medicine based on scientific evidence. How will you know if this is the case with your physicians? Ask them for the scientific basis for a specific recommendation. Many patients are wary that their physician will be offended by their questions. However, your peace of mind depends upon feeling confident about the treatment recommended. If the doctor seems threatened by your questions, beware. A knowledgeable and caring physician will not hesitate to explain the basis for a recommendation.

Getting a Second Opinion

You will begin by meeting with the initial consulting oncologist. Whether you are referred to the consulting oncologist by your diagnosing radiologist, by an ob-gyn, or by a surgeon, the first oncological opinion will map out an initial treatment plan. This is by no means a *final* treatment plan or the only treatment plan. You needn't feel disloyal in seeking another opinion, since a second opinion can bring added comfort and security. In the rare circumstance in which two oncologists differ dramatically as to the recommended treatment, you can only benefit from having two knowledgeable professionals discuss your case and, in most situations, resolve their differences. These differences, when explained to the patient, often stimulate a dialogue and, ultimately, a deeper understanding of the recommended treatment.

Getting a second opinion necessitates the assistance of the consulting physician's office staff in gathering records, slides, and films. You may need to pick up the material personally and deliver it, either by hand or by mail, to the institution you'll be visiting for the second opinion. It is critical that your biopsy slides and mammograms and/or ultrasound films be reviewed by the consulting team prior to your meeting. Your biopsy slides should be officially reviewed by an outside pathologist who has a specialization in breast pathology. A review of your mammograms is also important, and this should include the uninvolved breast. Fewer than 10 percent of women have problems in both breasts, but it is very important, if this is the case, to recognize it early, because it will affect decisions about your treatment. When you inquire about the consultation, determine if you will receive a formal report on the review of your slides and films. If your initial consulting oncologists have agreed to stay involved, then results and reports from the outside review should be sent to them on your request. Ideally, your primary treating doctor(s) will be in the loop; but it is you, the patient, who is instigating this review, and you should be treated with the same respect a physician gives a colleague, with copies of all reports coming directly to you.

A list of potential sources for a second opinion is included in the Resources section at the back of this book. National Cancer Institute (NCI)–sponsored comprehensive cancer centers have second opinion services. Major universities with medical schools are also good sources. Many of the larger hospitals have a breast cancer center that offers second opinion services. It is important to ask if there is a formal program or system in place that facilitates the second opinion process.

Preparation for your consultation is your responsibility as well as the consulting physician's. The basic guidelines for a second opinion are:

1. Inform your primary physician and/or your diagnosing physician that you plan to seek another opinion.
2. Ask for his/her help in suggesting a facility and getting your records and material ready to bring to the second facility.

3. Select a doctor, breast cancer center, or hospital to approach. Organizations such as the American Cancer Society, National Cancer Institute, and the Y-Me Support Group can also help provide second opinion sites. Would you feel more comfortable going out of town or staying local for your second opinion? Out-of-town opinions are sometimes less threatening to your home treatment team.

4. Contact the facility you have selected for the second opinion. Obtain a detailed list of the information it requires and the contact person or coordinator with whom you will be working and to whom you should direct both your questions and the materials, once obtained.

5. Be clear with the facility that you are making an appointment for a second opinion only, not to follow up for treatment. Although you may eventually choose to use this facility, you want an unbiased opinion, not an opinion that might be influenced by the consulting professionals' desire and/or expectation that you will be their patient.

6. Make sure you are receiving accurate information regarding your diagnosis and the best advice on treatment planning. "Is this the best treatment that exists for my disease? Would your recommendation be any different if I had different insurance or an unlimited ability to pay for treatment out of pocket?"

7. Be prepared for the second opinion outcome by educating yourself, to the best of your ability, prior to the appointment, about your particular breast cancer.

8. Check with your insurance provider to confirm the availability of, and limitations of, benefits for a second opinion, including medical oncology, pathology, surgery and radiology.*

---

*For a more complete discussion of getting a second opinion, see *The Breast Cancer Survival Manual.*

A widely accepted myth is that HMOs will not pay for an outside second opinion. This is not true, as recent legislation has mandated that HMOs must cover the cost of second opinions. Many HMOs have contracted with outside institutions to perform this service. If you are a member of an HMO, you will need to contact its member services department and inquire as to the process of authorizing second opinions. Regardless of whether you are covered by an HMO or not, it is a good idea to confirm the availability of insurance benefits.

Getting the Results

Although I have made my case for pursuing a second opinion, I understand that it is often anxiety provoking to delay beginning treatment while you wait for this opinion. Most major treatment centers understand the urgency and will see you within a few days to a week. It will take some time to gather your materials, which, ideally, have been reviewed prior to your appointment. During this time, if you feel confident and comfortable with the original treatment plan, physician, and facility that has been recommended, you can proceed with the scheduling of the proposed treatment. It can always be canceled or modified, depending on new knowledge you may receive from the outside review.

Because the information you'll receive in the second opinion will often be highly technical and emotional for you, it is important to bring a companion with you for the appointment. A tremendous amount of information will be covered, and a second set of ears can help you keep track so that no important details are missed. Be sure that both you and your companion take notes and ask questions about anything you don't understand. Many physicians provide a tape recording of the session for the patient to take home to review or allow others to hear the session. You might consider asking if there will be any objection to your bringing a tape recorder to the meeting. Given the intense level of information and emotions evoked, the tape is a helpful resource, and usually it will not offend the physician if you request to tape the session. If there is an objection, once again, beware.

Occasionally the reviewing physicians disagree significantly with the primary oncologic treatment plan. What then? It's always reassuring to get confirmation that the first opinion is accurate and correct, but if there is a difference of opinion, it is critical to question why. What difference would the change in treatment make? What are the clinical data to support this conflicting recommendation? Unfortunately, there can be some showmanship in these second opinion sessions. There can also be an attitude of superiority, most commonly experienced at academic institutions where prejudice against "local medical doctors," often referred to as LMDs, is not uncommon. The ultimate goal is to promote optimal patient care through the reconciling of differences and the affirmation of consistencies in treatment recommendations.

Every physician, no matter how geographically remote his or her practice is, has the opportunity to stay current. The real issue is whether the physician has made the effort to be in contact with colleagues and therefore has a team that he or she communicates with and that will work together. In my sister's case, I did not believe her physicians were current, nor was there a collaborative program in place. In breast cancer, the creation of a collaborative approach is extremely labor-intensive and, to be cost-effective, requires a certain volume of women being diagnosed with the disease who are requesting this service. Thus it is reasonable for you to ask how many breast cancer patients a physician or an institution treats in any given year. There is no one answer to this question that should make you feel comfortable, but for an institution that treats breast cancer patients, two cases a week or one hundred cases per year should be the minimal requirement.

It is not critical that you have a surgeon or oncologist who treats only breast cancer. The disease is, unfortunately, prevalent enough that general surgeons and oncologists can have plenty of experience.

In some practices or geographic areas, dedicated breast specialists could not survive financially. The truth is that insurance reimbursement for breast surgery is inadequate, particularly if the surgeon takes care to do an optimal procedure with a good cosmetic result. Physicians who do a really good job in breast cancer treatment have a passion for it; their financial gain is always secondary.

Proceeding with Treatment

⬥ Once you feel you have a consensus regarding your particular breast cancer and the recommended treatment before you, the next step is to proceed with treatment. Breast cancer treatment always requires *local control*, which entails removing the tumor completely from the breast. When, based upon an assessment of the tumor size and its nature, there is a significant likelihood that single cells may have migrated away from the breast into your lymph system or blood, systemic treatment—either chemotherapy or hormonal therapy—is appropriate. The usual sequence of treatment is local surgical treatment first, followed by systemic treatment.

However, recently this sequence has been reversed in situations where it is known that the patient will require systemic treatment and when the size of the tumor at diagnosis would normally dictate that a mastectomy would be recommended. It is now possible to obtain tremendous information about the cancer from a small, core biopsy of breast tissue, about the size of a pencil lead. This biopsy information, along with the imaging and knowing the physical size of the tumor, can determine if systemic therapy is necessary. It is important to ask whether and to what extent you will benefit from systemic therapy, since initiating it before surgery might cause the tumor to shrink in a manner that would allow greater choice in local surgical control, that is, a wide local excision or lumpectomy rather than a mastectomy.

Another question often addressed in treatment plans involves lymph node removal. Whether a cancer has spread to the lymph system has, traditionally, been critical in deciding if chemotherapy is necessary and to what extent. Newer imaging techniques and new methods of locating the first draining or sentinel node are alleviating the need for a full lymph node removal in many cases. Treatment timing, sequencing, and lymph node dissection are areas of debate among breast cancer specialists and are indicative of how state-of-the-art treatment is changing.

There is no question that being well informed, prepared, and aware prior to choosing a treating medical team and deciding on a treatment plan is the greatest step toward receiving superior care. Understanding the nature of your tumor allows you to pursue treatment that is tailored to you and your cancer. Knowledge of the sociopolitical forces at work in medicine and knowledge of the individual physicians participating in your care allow you to ask informed questions. The answers will reconfirm your confidence in the competence of your caregivers and make the treatment not something that is simply done to you, but something done with your full and free endorsement.

Do your homework. Make sure you're on the right track and *move forward.*

≈ 4 ≈

Treating the Whole Woman

If our healers . . . can keep open-minded, if they can practice the healing arts with compassion, skill, and mindful-
ness, and, most important, if they can treat the spirit as well
as the body, then we can truly enjoy optimal health.
—Brian Weiss, M.D., author of
Message from the Masters

Increasing specialization in medicine means that doctors more and
more frequently treat only one part of the body. There is also a tendency to focus on the immediate physical crisis and a failure to address
the context in which the crisis has occurred. This context is not just
the whole body—it is the whole person. For many physicians, it is
sometimes easier to deal with a damaged brain, a blocked artery, or a
diseased breast than it is to deal with a whole complex human being
whose survival may now depend on their care. For me, this is what
makes being a doctor such a fulfilling, rich, and fascinating profession—to be able to intervene in another human being's life, in this
crucible we call illness, and make a difference.

The managed care system also dehumanizes the patient, but for altogether different and more frightening reasons; specifically, it views each
patient as a potential financial liability. The more health problems

identified, the costlier the care. In the managed care model, potential patients are referred to as "lives," as if they were expendable units to be traded as commodities. Newspapers commonly report that "X" HMO has become insolvent and "Y" HMO will take over its 10,000 "lives." This reflects the extent to which the dehumanization has permeated our society—even our newspapers have adopted the language.

It goes without saying that human beings need to treat one another with respect and dignity. Although we are all accountable to this standard, physicians must be even more so because of the nature of their work. But their responsibilities go beyond mere respect and dignity. Healing illness is a complex process that is dependent upon the interaction between a person who has a disease and a person who is designated to relieve or eliminate the disease, the healer. Whatever the cause, illness is a life experience, and it contains an opportunity for growth.

I have likened illness to a crucible. A crucible is by definition a container in which change occurs. You, the patient, will ultimately determine whether or not the changes that occur as a result of your breast cancer experience are life-enhancing or life-diminishing. Your physician and treatment team are just one of many catalytic factors that contribute to creating an environment in which healing may occur. If your physician/healer shirks this duty of treating your breast cancer in the context of your whole being, this opportunity may be lost. You could not control whether or not your body developed cancer. You can, however, control whether or not you emerge richer from the experience.

Obviously your physician is not the sole healer in this process. You play a major role, but there are other important people who can help you. In my own practice, I have assembled a team of healers who work with me: physicians, nurses, researchers, medical assistants, and patient-care coordinators, as well as a psychotherapist, social worker, nutritionist, acupuncturist, and herbalist. Together, we work toward the common goal of healing. Every individual on the team, seen and unseen, professional, technical, or clerical, makes a contribution to the patient's care. Healing occurs at multiple levels, and no level should be overlooked. Ultimately, the healing team is not defined by the physician, but rather by the patient.

Each human being is an integrated complex organism in which the systems are interdependent. How foolish to unblock a clogged artery without addressing the underlying causes or to repair an unexplainable bone fracture without looking at the health of the entire skeleton. A physician can intervene or interpret a disease process, yet if the whole person is not addressed, including his or her emotional, mental, and spiritual well-being, we will never be true healers. From my patients I have learned this valuable lesson.

In 1997, I had the opportunity to offer a second opinion to a fifty-six-year-old Hindu woman. Originally diagnosed with breast cancer in 1985, Geeta had been fighting metastatic disease to her bone since 1989. In the process she had endured a mastectomy and an unsuccessful orthopedic surgery to stabilize her spine, as well as radiation therapy and a number of chemotherapies. She lived in constant back pain from the two rods that had been inserted along her spine to stabilize her vertebral column. As I reviewed her records in preparation for our meeting, I noticed her original physician's note at the time of her mastectomy. Her physician, though clearly desirous of giving her appropriate care, revealed much about his approach to her in this note. He said that she was emotionally depressed and anxious, and that she had "emotional problems dealing with this even prior to biopsy." He further described her as "extremely apprehensive and extremely difficult; both she and her family have a naturopathic background and conflicts with traditional medicine." He interpreted her distress about her limited range of motion post-mastectomy as an expression of her anxiety. He referred her for a mental health follow-up. She left this physician's care fairly rapidly and sought treatment from another Western-trained physician, who approached her disease using hormonal agents and radiation therapy, and then progressed to chemotherapy. I had undergone my medical training with her second physician and knew him to be an excellent clinician and a caring man. She had been quite satisfied with his care.

When I met Geeta, she was seeking a second opinion, but she was also interested in finding a physician closer to her home. She had lived with breast cancer and chronic pain for eight years by the time we met. I could see in her a quiet yet steely resolve as she and her family asked me questions about my philosophy of treatment and explained that she needed to feel in charge of her treatment. Though in significant pain, she managed to function by taking a painkiller each day and an occasional tranquilizer to enable her to rest. She had, at that time, active disease, and she allowed me to participate in her care.

She knew, from her back surgery, that the treatment might have lasting secondary effects that would dramatically impact her quality of life. She was determined to make informed decisions and to get answers to the questions she needed to ask. She asked them, thoughtfully and methodically. I knew that after each office visit there would be a call from her to verify her understanding about what we discussed, and to ask about other options. In each call she used her voice and will to make the treatment hers. Her husband, who accompanied her to virtually every office visit and treatment, referred to her as "The Boss." He supported her in her decision making, even when his feelings about the appropriate treatment differed from hers. She was a well-educated woman from a well-educated family. As a gifted writer and poet, she understood when she had been heard and when she had not; when she felt received as a self-determining human being and when she felt dismissed. It was clear that she would trust my judgment if she felt she could trust me as a person who would hold her welfare and beliefs in my heart and soul as well as my mind.

For the next few years, her disease ebbed and flowed. Eventually, the cancer spread to her liver. We exhausted virtually every available treatment. Her body could not tolerate more. So we waited. Unsure whether her body would rally or her disease relent, we watched and searched for new treatment. Still managing her pain as before, she declined additional pain medicines. Although I knew that she must be in tremendous pain, she continued on. If she was unable to tolerate more treatment, we knew that she would soon die. Her sister and brother-in-law, her beloved son, and her husband stood steadfastly by her, supporting her dignity always, letting her control her destiny. We were able to relieve some of her pain by removing the fluid from her abdomen that put pressure on her liver and spine. She did not speak of death, though she understood that she would die without further treatment. Each time I visited her she would say, "How are you doing, Dr. Link?" She never failed to acknowledge her caregivers or the importance of their lives even as she fought for her own.

I longed for Geeta to be free from pain, as I'm sure she did. However, it became apparent that she valued something else more, that she would be voting against the gift of life if she received medications that would stress her liver but relieve her of pain. For her, hospice care meant that she had rejected life; it was a move actively toward death. Her faith required that she lift up her soul to her god and receive his will. At the time, I was aware only of her need to be respected in her decision making. She did not speak of the beliefs that dictated her decision making, but I knew from her insistence how very important it was for me to support her *as she wished*.

Though practically hospice might have relieved much of her suffering, she was adamant that she did not want it involved. Her family honored that wish—until one Sunday. Watching her in pain, they decided that they would agree to have a hospice agency come to assess her. She died an hour before the hospice caseworker arrived.

Since her death, I have had many opportunities to think and feel about Geeta and her family. She did it her way—from the first moment of our healing relationship. She loved life and lived it fully and with dignity. She knew we loved her and wanted her to have a long and healthy life. And she maintained her integrity and her vote. We might advise, but she would decide.

Geeta's lesson is an important one. She teaches us that each of us has our own beliefs and philosophy about how we want to live and be treated. Your illness and treatment must fit into the fabric and the context of who you are. In this way, you have the opportunity to be the hero of your own life.

❧ 5 ❧

Your Doctor Is Human, Too

It takes two to speak truth—one to speak and another to hear.

—Henry David Thoreau

In the last chapter, I discussed the factors that influence your ability to trust your physician. Specifically, trust is enhanced by having a physician who is knowledgeable, committed to lifelong learning, and is comfortable educating you by responding to your questions. Developing trust between you and your physician requires a delicate balance of knowledge and compassion, communication, and experience. However, it requires even more than that.

I have already addressed your right to insist upon being treated and related to as a whole person. What I left out is how very important it is for you to relate to your physician as a whole person—with his or her own vast repertoire of life experiences. Your physicians may never choose to share with you their personal or private thoughts on their careers, but know that the decision to become involved in oncology was never casual. At some point in their careers all "cancer doctors"—be they medical oncologists, surgeons, radiation oncologists, or mammography-dedicated radiologists—have had to reckon with their own feelings of vulnerability, and fears of loss and failure. Cancer raises the specter of death, and death is the ultimate symbol of a physician's limitations.

It is important to remember this when you feel a loss of connection with your doctor. We physicians are people, too—with our own opportunities to learn and understand our limitations. Our responsibility to you is not to allow our personal issues and growth points to inappropriately affect your care.

This is a difficult chapter for me to write because it requires some self-exploration regarding my own feelings about medicine and being a physician. I must admit that writing it is somewhat cathartic, but my true purpose is to help you understand healing from the physician's perspective. I believe that almost all doctors are well-intentioned and have their patients' best interests at heart. In spite of this, I feel that a majority of women do not receive optimal breast cancer care in this country, and their doctors must bear a significant amount of the responsibility. There are a number of reasons for this, some of which I have already discussed, others I will now develop. The major contributors are burnout, ignorance, ego, and denial of our own vulnerability.

Physicians begin their careers as medical students—young men and women who have chosen a career in healing—and it is interesting to understand what motivates a young physician to go into a particular field of study. In my own education, there was a point when I thought I could never go into medicine. In high school I was a runner, and I received a scholarship to USC to run on the track team. As an undergraduate, I was a premed student like 40 percent of the students at that time. My track coach at USC, Willie Wilson, was like a second father to me. During my sophomore year, when he was forty years old, Willie was diagnosed with terminal cancer. I was devastated by his illness. I sympathized to such a degree that I almost dropped out of school. I couldn't express to him how much I cared and what he meant to me. I was unable to concentrate and I began having difficulty sleeping.

Willie Wilson was a fantastic coach and a wonderful human being.

A tribute to his coaching was that we had the best track team in the country. I was one of several middle-distance runners on the team and, together with three of my teammates, decided to attempt to break the world record in the two-mile relay and dedicate the record to our coach before he died. Interestingly, as we pursued the record, the support of my teammates and the focus of working toward this goal brought me out of my depression. I believe that if we had planned and done this for our own gratification, it would probably have been impossible. But because we so desperately wanted to give Coach Wilson a gift that would speak to him in the language he had used to teach us, through track, so much about life, character, and values, we were able to transcend our individual limits. For our beloved coach we were able "to go the distance," and we did, indeed, break the world record on a warm spring evening in 1966 at the Coliseum Relays. The following Sunday morning the *Los Angeles Times* ran a lead article about our accomplishment and our dedication of the record to Coach Wilson. He died two weeks later, but he was there to see us excel in his honor.

I dropped out of premed and switched to English literature. Because of my experience with my coach's illness, I could not imagine dealing with grief of such magnitude on a regular basis. It was a period in my life that allowed me to explore who I was and what I wanted to be. It was so gratifying to be able to read the classics that I hardly missed the science. However, I began to realize that what most compelled me in literature was the sense of life captured, and my ability to feel about those lives, albeit in a controlled or safe manner. Nowhere is the preciousness of life clearer than in medicine. I realized I was running away from a calling in medicine that might give me true professional and personal happiness, even though I did not know how to manage the emotions that medicine evoked. Many of the writers who had influenced me greatly were physicians, such as William Osler, one of the fathers of modern medicine, writing from their experiences as healers. I realized that leaving medicine might be the most regrettable step I could take, so during my senior year I carried three extra classes and completed my premed requirements.

I had recommitted to becoming a medical doctor, but I still had tremendous reservations about my ability to take care of sick human beings. What I didn't realize then, and learned later from my greatest teacher in medical school, was that one could be a healer and still be able to be empathic and feel compassion for another human being in distress. What I experienced with my coach was *sympathy*, which is a double burden—you feel another's suffering plus you anticipate your life without that person. *Empathy* allows you to separate yourself from another's suffering but at the same time have compassion for that individual's situation. If the person has a terminal disease, you can appreciate what the patient contributed to your own life and the lives of those he or she loves. Physicians must have the ability to empathize. If not, they will rapidly burn out. In a futile attempt to protect themselves from this profound experience of vulnerability, physicians adopt an unflappable façade, an exterior that provides an illusion of safety but that cannot protect their souls.

· · ·

It hasn't been easy, but the rewards have far outweighed the losses. I was privileged to learn this balance from wonderful teachers and role models. The most important teachers were the patients, who taught me humility and compassion as well as the complex ways in which human beings develop and respond to illness. To have the privilege of entering another's life in the crisis of illness and to make a difference has been incredibly fulfilling.

Early on in medical school, I had no intention of going into oncology. I still suffered tremendous heartache from my experience with my coach, and I covered the wound with denial and avoidance. At this point, I met an orthopedic surgeon who was my instructor in a course called "Introduction to Clinical Medicine" (ICM). Dr. Loren Stephens became my advisor and friend, and the most influential person in my development as a young physician. We had long discussions about becoming a doctor. He taught me about the complexity of human disease and the difference between curing and healing. He emphasized not to treat a symptom but to look at the entire person for the underlying cause. He said that illness creates the opportunity for change and growth and that part of being a physician is to help a patient realize this.

I told Dr. Stephens about my track coach's death, and he then taught me the difference between empathy and sympathy. I asked if one could learn to be a healer and have empathy or whether it was something you were born with. He said he believed that most great healers were born with a gift but that they never stopped learning.

After I had been under Dr. Stephens's wing for several months in ICM, he arranged for me to interview a patient, a forty-two-year-old man who had broken his femur bone due to a malignancy known as multiple myeloma. I learned that the malignancy formed tumors that dissolved the bones and made them more prone to fractures. The patient had terminal cancer. I became frightened that I might not be able to control my emotions to complete the interview. I spent over an hour with this man whose leg was connected to a pulley contraption with a sandbag hanging at the end of the bed. He was in some physical pain and, my fear aside, I didn't want to impose on him. As a first-year student, I felt like an impostor. To my surprise, I got through it. He talked with me about his life and how sad he was that he would not see his teenage children grow into adults, and that he would have to leave his wife at the very time she needed his help the most. I asked how he knew this, and he said the doctors had told him he could not be cured and would die within eighteen months. My heart ached for him, but I kept listening, focused on his pain, and was able to continue.

I left that interview hurting, but it was different than it had been with Coach Wilson. This time, I understood that I could directly influence this patient's immediate quality of life simply by listening to his story, even if I could not alter his prognosis. He thanked me for listening, and he called me "Doctor." At that point I knew I could really be a doctor and I could take care of people who might die—that I did have the ability to manage my own feelings without losing them. This was the first of a number of patient interactions in my training that led me into the field of oncology.

As you proceed with your breast cancer journey, you will encounter a number of health care professionals who may seem insensitive and uncaring. In chapter 1, I mentioned the oncologist my mother first saw in the HMO, who communicated as if she were reading from a script, emotionless and matter-of-fact? Some physicians have difficulty balancing empathy and sympathy. It is impossible to remain sympathetic, aware of your own loss, and be effective as a healer—it is too painful— so the healer must assume other coping mechanisms. Ideally, the physician can focus on empathy and remain sensitive to the patient's feelings and needs. Under stress, less effective styles for healing may emerge that allow the healer to function, though less than optimally. He or she may become mechanical in behavior without feelings or emotion. Even worse, a physician may become angry and impatient with the very person he or she is attempting to help. I believe that this response is a protective mechanism. Being fully receptive to another human being is an art. That art is undercut by the necessities of heavy patient loads, intense patient needs, and insufficient time and energy to renew self. While these factors may explain inappropriate physician responses, there is no excuse for them. As a patient you must be confident that you can speak directly to your doctor when you feel you have not been heard or have been dealt with inappropriately.

There are ways to initiate and promote a good reception. Simple questions that give the physician feedback about his or her demeanor often stimulate greater awareness and authenticity. Most physicians are responsive when they recognize that they have been inappropriate or nonempathic in their responses. If you find yourself on the receiving end of this type of behavior, remember that you are dealing with a human being first, and a physician second. Assume that this behavior is not a measure of how your physician regards you and your illness. If this is unusual behavior, it is quite likely that this individual is stressed or emotionally depleted and that your next encounter with him or her may be very different. These behaviors are much more common in medical systems where physicians feel ineffective due to insufficient time, insufficient resources, or lack of positive results from their efforts. Changing health care providers is always an option if you are consistently unable to receive the type of empathic, supportive healing environment you need. However, no one wants to leave a physician who has been significantly involved in her treatment.

Furthermore, physicians generally don't want to lose patients due to a perception of physician insensitivity or loss of connection. As human beings and as doctors, this represents a personal failure. Because this is true, most doctors will respond to a calm yet direct inquiry such as, "Doctor, you seem to have a lot on your mind today. Is there anything you are concerned about in my care that you are not feeling comfortable about? I don't want to leave today worried that there is something crucial you haven't told me. I'm concerned because you seem different than you have in our past meetings. Are you okay?" Most physicians upon hearing this kind of statement understand that their demeanor has changed and is distressing you. Their response should be taken at face value. However, if your physician is not being authentic in his or her responses, you will have this experience frequently and will want to review the benefits of this very important treatment relationship. You will have this relationship long after treatment is complete as you return for checkups and ongoing breast cancer surveillance. You need to feel comfortable and understood. Your physician needs to be of service to you, to facilitate your survival and quality of life. It is this commitment that took this doctor into oncology in the first place. It takes the compassionate understanding of both you and your physician to create a lasting, healing relationship.

❧ 6 ❧

Survival

Even if I knew that tomorrow the world would go to pieces,
I would still plant my apple tree.
                                        —Martin Luther King, Jr.

Survival is defined as "continuing to live." All women survive, or
continue to live, after their initial diagnosis of breast cancer in spite of
negative thoughts and bad dreams. Two factors are especially important after hearing the diagnosis; the first has to do with cure—or
disease-free survival—and the second, and arguably the more important, is quality of life after diagnosis. The good news is that increasing
numbers of women survive breast cancer and ultimately will die of an
unrelated cause. Keep in mind that heart disease kills far more women
than breast cancer does. Approximately 80 percent of women today
are cured of breast cancer, meaning that they live the rest of their lives
without a recurrence. You want to be in this group.

In order to maximize your chances of cure and survival, you need
to make an objective assessment of your risk of not surviving breast
cancer. Given your personal and family history, what are the most
probable health problems you're likely to face? I believe, first and foremost, that you should consider the most up-to-date treatment options
that modern medicine has to offer. This may involve participating

in a clinical trial of a new drug or even using a promising new treatment that is being researched. You may want to consider "alternative" therapies—not as an alternative to traditional medicine but as an adjunct to what has been scientifically proven to be helpful. At our breast cancer center, we commonly refer patients for a consult with an acupuncturist to assist with nausea management, in addition to the traditional anti-nausea drug regimen. Let your team know what you are interested in while you're actively in treatment as well as afterward so they can make appropriate referrals. Your caregivers should communicate with one another to create a unified treatment plan. Once treatment has been completed and you have given yourself the best chance of cure, you must go forward with your life.

A few years ago, I took care of a woman named Alice who had newly diagnosed breast cancer. Together we developed a comprehensive treatment plan that gave her an excellent chance of survival. She received a wide local excision of the primary tumor with a sentinel lymph node sampling, six months of chemotherapy followed by radiation for approximately six weeks, and then took an oral medication, tamoxifen, for five years. She did relatively well during the active phases of the treatment: surgery, chemo, and radiation. But once she completed this active treatment, she went into a fearful, anxiety-dominated depression. Alice was forty-six years old, and though recovered from her treatment and in excellent physical health, she was sure her life was over, that she was dying of breast cancer. I treated her with several antidepressant drugs with little success, and I then referred her to a psychiatrist. Nothing seemed to help much. She became fixated on making the five-year anniversary without relapse. I suspected that was because her mother had had breast cancer, had relapsed after four years, and ultimately died of the disease.

As Alice waited for the five-year mark, it seemed that she almost stopped living. She developed an almost superstitious quiet. It seemed as if she was afraid to do anything lest it somehow provoke a recurrence. She dropped out of all her social activities. She had divorced ten years before her diagnosis and had been involved with a very supportive man. After she was diagnosed, she ended the relationship. Her two grown children lived far away and were not aware of how the cancer had altered her life, which was now consumed by her health concerns and her fear of relapse. I encouraged her to get involved in support groups, but she refused. She became more withdrawn and reclusive, and her two children came to see me out of concern for their mother. I explained that she had an excellent chance of being cured and that I was worried about her inability to live life more fully. For many patients, the close encounter with the reality of death that the experience of breast cancer forces upon them also results in a profound commitment to live life to its fullest. These patients don't just survive, they thrive. They insist on it. They have fought so hard for the quantity of their lives that they insist the quality be the best. Not so for Alice. She was almost fifty years old and she was consumed by depression and anxiety. At some point I suggested she get a dog or some type of pet to encourage her in investing in a relationship. She did get a small dog, which seemed to ease her loneliness and bring her joy.

On her fifth anniversary, she came to the office and we gave her a small party to celebrate the milestone. She told us that she was feeling more optimistic about the future and that she was ready to really start living again. The following week she had a massive cerebral hemorrhage. She died three days later. Her children requested a postmortem examination. No evidence of breast cancer was found.

The story of Alice, as sad as it is, holds an important lesson for us. Life is precious and short. Once a diagnosis is made and optimal treatment has occurred, you return from the strange journey of treatment to a life renewed—another chance to begin. Though no one can guarantee cure, you choose where you will focus your mind and heart. As strange as it may sound, for many survivors, breast cancer is a gift that can enhance the rest of their lives. Once you have knowledge of your breast cancer risk/potential for cure, based on the current research, you are empowered to make decisions as to the role this information will play in your life.

Assessing the Probability of Cure

⊙ The first step in the pursuit of quality of life is to give yourself the best chance of disease-free survival. To do this, you need an accurate assessment of your chance of being cured. This assessment is based on the characteristics of the cancer: both the degree of malignancy and the extent of disease. You need to be apprised of your risk of cells having escaped through the bloodstream to another part of your body (systemic spread). We hope soon to have an accurate test that will indicate systemic spread. We know that fast-growing, aggressive breast cancers, if they relapse systemically, will do so much sooner than slow-growing, indolent types of breast cancer. The problem is that it probably takes very few escaped cells to cause relapse, and no test can show minimal microscopic disease with accuracy. Certainly no scan can show minimal disease. Our hope is to find an abnormal protein that is shed into the bloodstream—something akin to the PSA in prostate cancer. However, breast cancer is much more heterogeneous than prostate cancer. Until we have such a test, we must rely on the specific pathology of the tumor, lymph node status, and blood markers to assess the likelihood of systemic spread.

Once you know your risk of systemic spread, you then need to be informed as to what can be done to improve your chance of cure and at what cost to you—not financial cost, but cost to your quality of life. You must always remember that this risk assessment is a statistical analysis based on thousands of women who have preceded you in this battle. What happens to you is unique, and there is no way to know with certainty what will happen in your particular case with or without further treatment.

The first doctor many women with newly diagnosed breast cancer see is the general surgeon. While general surgeons may be able to accurately assess systemic risk, they are often concerned first and foremost about surgically controlling the cancer. A medical oncologist deals with the larger picture of cancer, its biology and natural history. Additionally, in order to assess systemic risk accurately, the pathologist should have an adequate sample of the cancer as well as a sampling of the draining lymph nodes. This usually requires the surgeon to operate prior to making a decision about systemic therapy. Occasionally, when a cancer has been proven through an ultrasound-guided needle biopsy, there may be enough information, based upon the size and pathology, to proceed with chemotherapy or a combination of chemo and hormonal therapy before the actual surgical procedure. When it is indicated, I am a proponent of this neo-adjuvant, or preoperative systemic therapy. There are a number of advantages for taking this approach:

1. It provides the opportunity to determine if the systemic therapy can kill the cancer. If we leave the primary breast cancer in place, we can determine if the chemo or hormonal therapy is working by observing the cancer's response—does it shrink, stay the same size, or grow? Periodic imaging during treatment provides us with this data. It makes sense that if the therapy works on the primary cancer, it should also work on any microscopic cells that have escaped to any location in the body.

2. It allows a better chance for breast conservation. Women with cancers too large to avoid mastectomy, if surgically treated before systemic treatment, may be good candidates for breast conservation after preoperative systemic therapy shrinks the tumor. The cosmetic result of breast-conserving surgery is usually better because less breast tissue needs to be removed.

3. Recent studies have shown that a significant number of women will have circulating cancer cells during and following their surgical procedure. Theoretically it should be safer to do the surgery after chemotherapy because the exposure to cytotoxic treatment alters the tumor cell, inhibiting the cancer's subsequent ability to establish itself at a metastatic site. The cancer cells are therefore less likely to take hold if they escape into the lymph or blood.

4. Women who have good responses to preoperative chemo/hormonal therapy have a very low systemic relapse rate. Women with complete disappearance of the primary cancer or conversion of involved lymph nodes to negative lymph nodes at the time of surgery have a very high cure rate.

5. Women who desire a mastectomy in spite of a good response to systemic therapy or who require mastectomy because of remaining ductal cancer in situ (DCIS) often can have immediate reconstruction, without concern about the healing problems secondary to chemotherapy.

The use of preoperative chemotherapy often depends on the surgeon's understanding and recognition of these advantages. Many general surgeons do not consider this approach because it is unfamiliar and outside of their area of specialization.

My sister's case (described in chapter 2) is an example of all of the above. In New Zealand, where she was diagnosed, physicians do not give chemotherapy prior to surgery except in the rare case of inflammatory breast cancer. My sister's tumor was amazingly responsive to preoperative chemo with conversion of multiple positive lymph nodes to negative status and complete disappearance of all invasive cancer. She still required a mastectomy because she had extensive in situ disease that usually doesn't respond to chemotherapy. But we were able to learn that her cancer was responsive to the chemo she received, and because of the complete disappearance of the invasive cancer after chemotherapy, she has a very good statistical chance of being cured. If she had had the mastectomy first, we would not have been able to obtain this valuable information, and we would have had the added concern that the surgery was occurring at a time when the cancer was advancing.

Disease-free survival is our goal. But how does a woman know for sure that she is cured? For those women with invasive breast cancer, nothing is absolute. Even women with the smallest cancers have a slight risk of systemic relapse in spite of the most aggressive treatment. However, the fact that there is a small gray cloud in the sky doesn't mean it's going to rain.

For those with bigger clouds—women whose draining lymph nodes contain cancer or who have large tumors—relapse is not a given or inevitable. I care for a significant number of women who were told that they almost certainly would relapse, but they return year after year to tell me about their disease-free and joy-filled lives. After breast cancer, there can be a reflex panic brought to the surface by some seemingly insignificant event. This can happen with a new ache or pain or when an abnormal blood test brings up the fear of recurrence. As stated previously, and I cannot reiterate it enough, I believe that once treatment has been completed, you need to assume that you are cured and live life to the fullest. Those fleeting reminders should stimulate you to refocus on what is important to you.

Assessing Quality of Life

As time passes, the anxiety over the possibility of a recurrence naturally lessens. Unfortunately, there is no cutoff time when recurrence is no longer possible. Alice said she was going to go on with her life after five years, but there is nothing magical about five years. The lesson, not only for breast cancer survivors but for every one of us, is: *Don't put your life on hold. Rather, hold on to your life.* Since a majority of women will experience disease-free survival, a major concern is the quality of life. Most of us want more than mere survival. Freud identified the primary needs of human beings as the need to love and to engage in meaningful work. As I observe my patients, I see the potency of the need to love and be loved *now*, not in some distant someday. I also notice that survivors who are most fulfilled, by their own report, are those who have learned to approach their lives informed but not obsessed by a profound awareness of the preciousness of life.

Vital in the quality of life assessment is knowing the risks and benefits of replacement hormones following breast cancer treatment. We know that estrogen powerfully affects a woman's health and vitality. Estrogen helps to maintain vaginal lubrication, bladder control, bone density, cardiovascular health, and, to some extent, mental functioning. The cardiovascular benefit has recently been challenged by newer studies. It may be that the progesterone added to estrogen replacement may diminish the benefit of estrogen. Yet postmenopausal women on hormone replacement therapy are almost always immediately taken off it when they are diagnosed with breast cancer. In addition, a new class of drugs known as aromatase inhibitors, used to treat certain types of breast cancer, completely shut down even the minimal amount of estrogen produced in a postmenopausal woman's body. At this time, we don't know what the long-term effects of this total reduction in estrogen will be, but clinical trials have already shown that short-term side effects include hot flashes, painful intercourse, and an increased likelihood of urinary tract infection. There is concern over possible diminished cognitive functioning and loss of bone density, but we will learn more as trials of these drugs continue.

To take or not to take replacement hormones is a dilemma for every woman, regardless of whether she has had breast cancer. On the one hand, estrogen exposure increases risk of breast cancer; on the other, estrogen makes women feel better and function better. This complex issue is especially poignant for breast cancer survivors, who seem to be in a "damned if you do, damned if you don't" position. You'll need to discuss this issue thoroughly with your physician. In making a decision, both you and your doctor need to consider your particular situation and needs. (This subject will be addressed in more detail in chapter 14.)

As in all treatment, you and your oncologist will assess the risks and benefits of a variety of treatments. Ultimately, you must make informed decisions that make the most sense to you based upon your unique situation at the time of diagnosis—and then not second-guess yourself. It is certain that the science of breast cancer will change in time and that your situation will, in the future, be treated differently. We must do the best we can *now*.

☙ 7 ☙

Saving Your Breast

I learned that there are troubles of more than one kind.
Some come from ahead and some from behind.

—Dr. Seuss

After "Will I survive?" the most frequent question women diagnosed with breast cancer ask is "What will happen to my breast?" Many women are haunted by the memory of a mother's or a grandmother's mastectomy scar. The truth is that in the first eighty years of the last century, breast cancer was treated almost solely by male surgeons with almost total disregard for a woman's appearance, body image, or feelings.

Breast surgery consists of two basic choices: The first option is breast-conserving surgery, which is removal of the cancerous tissue and sufficient surrounding tissue (margins) to ensure that the remaining breast tissue has no residual tumor. This is known as a lumpectomy or wide local excision. The second option is mastectomy, which is a total removal of the breast tissue, nipple and areola, as well as skin. Fortunately, today a majority of women can achieve local control of their disease by having breast-conserving surgery with an excellent cosmetic result. In our centers, approximately 80 percent of women undergo limited surgery with breast conservation, followed by radiation therapy. In this type of surgery there are usually two small scars (one on the breast and the other under the arm) with some mild skin changes following radiation (see figure 7.1). It is especially difficult to achieve good cosmetic results in women who have large cancers and small breast size and in women with cancers that are located in the medial (middle) or lower aspect of the breast. Our surgeons try to give the best cosmetic result possible without compromising local control. Often they will move normal tissue to fill in a defect created by the excision of the affected area. Some women are unpredictably sensitive to radiation and will develop shrinkage of the breast and thickening of the remaining breast tissue over time. In my experience, however, this is rare.

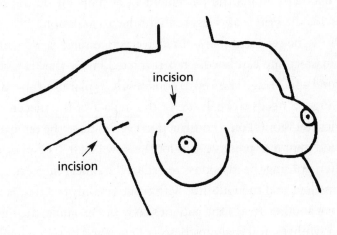

FIGURE 7.1

Additionally, women who have cancers with an associated ductal cancer in situ (DCIS) component involving a large area of the breast duct system require large amounts of tissue to be removed. This can lead to a dissatisfying cosmetic result. Lobular cancers, which occur in the breast lobule as opposed to the duct, often involve larger areas than we actually see on a mammogram or feel in a clinical exam. This frequently requires larger amounts of tissue to be removed to ensure that the cancer-involved breast tissue has been completely removed—referred to as "clearing the margins." There are situations in which breast conservation is possible but produces inferior cosmetic results. In a case like this, mastectomy and the newer reconstruction techniques will usually give superior results and eliminate the need for radiation.

If, for example, a quarter of the breast needs to be removed, the cosmetic result is usually significantly affected. However, for some women, a better cosmetic result is achieved by a mastectomy with reconstruction if the decision is made prior to beginning radiation. Once radiation is added to surgery, there may be some further shrinkage and fibrosis (thickening) as the fluid-filled cavity shrinks. This process distinctly limits the placement of an implant during reconstruction, as the skin is also less resilient due to radiation.

With the newer techniques of reconstructive surgery, women who require mastectomy can have a reconstructed breast that is aesthetic and natural appearing. The key to good results is planning ahead. The cancer surgeon needs to be aware of the impact of the placement of the surgical incision(s) on reconstruction even as he or she removes the cancer and must also preserve skin for the new breast. The plastic surgeon, often utilizing the incisions created by the cancer surgeon, creates a skin envelope and then fills this with tissue (mainly fat) that is transferred from another area of the patient's body (for example, the tummy) or with a synthetic internal prosthesis (silicone and/or saline implant).

Women with large amounts of DCIS (ductal carcinoma in situ) or women with lobular-type breast cancer should prepare for possible mastectomy. The goal is to get a one-centimeter clear margin all around the cancer. Both extensive DCIS and infiltrating lobular cancer make it difficult, though, to get this clear margin and still leave enough breast tissue to give a good cosmetic result. In addition, with infiltrating lobular cancer it is important to address the fact that there is an increased risk of an occurrence of another cancer in the presently unaffected breast or later in the treated breast. Some women consider bilateral mastectomy and reconstruction at the same time. Although this involves the possible loss of a currently uninvolved breast, the likelihood of subsequent cancer over the woman's lifetime may be significant enough to justify removing the unaffected breast. Additionally, bilateral mastectomy allows women the increased potential of a cosmetically well-matched reconstruction.

In 1998, I treated a twenty-five-year-old woman who presented with an invasive lobular cancer. Given Kelly's age, the nature of her tumor, her desire to live a life free from the dread of an occurrence or reoccurrence of cancer in her breasts, and the limitations of mammography with lobular carcinoma, she made the very difficult decision to have bilateral mastectomies with reconstruction. Although she had always hoped to nourish her children through breast feeding, her experience with breast cancer at such an early age profoundly affected her. She had undergone aggressive chemotherapy and hoped to do everything possible to avoid a second breast cancer. Interestingly, her age, the nature of her tumor, and her surgeon's confidence in improved breast surveillance in the near future influenced him to recommend breast conservation. Kelly actually had to convince her surgeon that she fully understood her options and that she was making the best decision *for her*. With adequate information as to your options, you, too, must determine for yourself the intervention that will give you peace of mind as well as the best chance for a cure. Of significance in Kelly's decision was the opportunity to pursue bilateral reconstruction with a premier breast reconstructive surgeon. She had done her homework, understood her options, and had realistic expectations. She remains satisfied with her decision four years later. She continues to be disease-free and volunteers to meet with women considering the possibility of mastectomy. We find that it is very helpful for a woman thinking about a mastectomy with reconstruction to actually observe a woman who has had the procedure.

Occasionally women with an increased risk of breast cancer through heredity opt for the removal of both breasts, followed by immediate reconstruction, to prevent the likely occurrence of breast cancer. One such case I counseled was that of a thirty-four-year-old registered nurse named Mary Ellen, whose mother had died of breast cancer in her mid-thirties. At the time her mother died, Mary Ellen was only seven years old. Her mother's mother had also died of breast cancer in her forties. Breast cancer had been a legacy throughout her mother's side of the family. Recently one of her first cousins (her maternal uncle's daughter) had been diagnosed. Mary Ellen came to me for counseling regarding genetic testing, which I strongly recommended. She received approval from her insurance company, and we drew her blood and sent it to Myriad Genetic Laboratories in Utah, where most of the genetic testing for breast cancer is performed. Three weeks passed and we received a phone call that indeed Mary Ellen was BRCA2 positive. BRCA2 is one of the two genes that have been identified that give rise to breast cancer (the other gene is BRCA1). This meant that she had inherited a gene from her mother that gave her approximately a 70 percent chance of developing breast cancer over the next fifteen to twenty years. I met with Mary Ellen and her husband to discuss her options. The statistical probability of her developing breast cancer, her personal history of losing her mom to it at an early age, and the fact that she never even knew her maternal grandmother were key factors in her decision to have prophylactic mastectomies.

Mary Ellen was of Irish descent, thin, with a very light complexion. She had small breasts and used a padded bra to make them fuller in clothes. At times she had considered implants, but never pursued them because of her fears of developing breast cancer. She had suspected that at some point she might have to consider having her breasts removed. The positive gene test gave her the courage to proceed with mastectomies. She saw a breast surgeon and a plastic surgeon who does a large number of breast reconstructions. Together they planned bilateral skin-sparing mastectomies, with the placement of expanders beneath her pectoralis muscles. "Skin-sparing" means that very little skin is removed with the underlying glandular tissue. The incision removes the nipple and areola and leaves the inferior mammary fold that keeps the contour of the breast (see figure 7.2).

After the breast tissue is removed, an expandable implant is inserted behind the muscle. Following this procedure, it is filled with salt water to stretch the skin as well as the muscle, which acts like a sling with which to hold the implant. Mary Ellen decided that if she was going to go through with this, she might as well increase her breast size. This meant expanding the temporary implants several times before the permanent gel implants were placed. The first phase of the surgery involved the

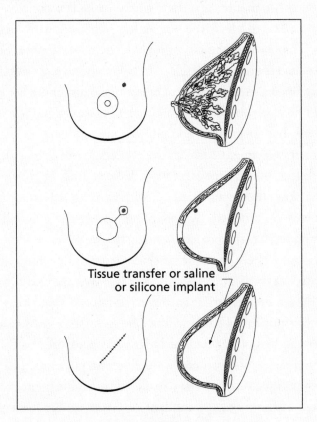

Tissue transfer or saline or silicone implant

FIGURE 7.2
Skin-sparing procedure (mastectomy)

removal of both breasts, including the nipples and areolas. The surgeon left thin skin flaps, and then the plastic surgeon inserted temporary expandable implants underneath her chest muscles. All of this was done as an outpatient. (Sometimes this procedure requires a one-night stay in the hospital.) Her breast tissue was sent to the lab for careful analysis and, to our surprise, there was a tiny, two-millimeter cancer sitting in the upper outer quadrant of her left breast. Fortunately at the stage it was discovered, it was highly curable with the surgery alone. When we met after surgery, I gave her the news. She broke down, sobbing with relief and gratitude that she would not follow her mother's fate.

Mary Ellen continued with the expansion of her expander implants over the next two months and then, when she had expanded to the size breasts she desired, had the expanders replaced with permanent implants. Through her choice of prophylactic mastectomies, her breast cancer risk had been greatly reduced to below the average woman's risk. There remained a small amount of breast tissue just under her skin, but this could be easily followed with clinical breast exams. She was very pleased with her appearance and allowed me to take a photo to show other women who might consider the procedure (see page 75).

Mary Ellen's breast removal scars were horizontal. Nipples were created using skin and tissue folded up, with cartilage added for firmness. The areolas were tattooed. By preserving most of the skin, particularly in the lower aspect, the procedure made the new breasts look natural.

The point of these examples is that a woman now has options for local control of the cancer; regardless of whether she chooses mastectomy or lesser surgery, she can have confidence that she will look good. This is not to say there will not be scars or loss of sensation, or grief over the loss of her natural breast, but compared to the recent past when a majority of women were given no alternative to a modified radical mastectomy, we have made considerable progress.

Progress in the surgical treatment of breast cancer has come as a result of the passionate interest of many significant people, who took it upon themselves to research and advocate for treatment options that

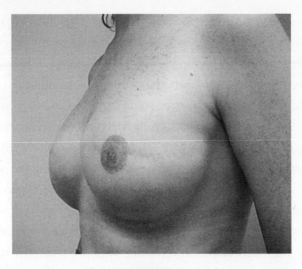

FIGURE 7.3

more fully addressed the whole woman. As recently as the 1980s, women had to prepare for "what if?" scenarios with each surgical biopsy. Even though the biopsy would prove benign 90 percent of the time, all women had to consent to an immediate mastectomy if it was malignant. There was no opportunity to learn the diagnosis and become educated about the available options. During that period, many women with fibrocystic breasts had multiple biopsies, which left their breasts with multiple scars. The "one-stage" mastectomy, as it was called, meant that a woman was put to sleep and the lump was removed and sent to pathology for analysis. The tissue would be rapidly frozen, and a thin sliver shaved off, mounted on a glass slide, and examined under a microscope. If the tissue specimen was benign, all was well and the wound was closed. On the other hand, if it was cancer, the surgeon would begin a radical or a modified radical mastectomy. The difference was that with a radical, the underlying chest wall muscles were removed. General surgeons were getting rich on breast biopsies. I remember hearing a surgeon brag that the female breast sent all five of his children to college and paid his mortgage as well. When we introduced nonsurgical needle biopsies done by radiologists at our center in Long Beach back in the early 1980s, the twenty-three male surgeons doing breast biopsies at the time were furious. The number of "benign" surgical breast biopsies dropped from several thousand a year to several hundred.

This shift in approach, from treating the woman as an onlooker to including her as a conscious decision maker in the process was the passionate concern of breast cancer advocate Rose Kushner, who was outraged by the manner in which women were treated. Rose researched whether or not it would somehow compromise the outcome if the process became a two-step procedure in order to obtain the woman's knowing consent. She discovered that surgeons could locally excise the tumor and then discuss the results with the patient without any major downside. At this time, in the late 1970s, studies were showing that breast-conserving surgery followed by local radiation provided equal survival benefit as well as local control, compared to mastectomy. Rose questioned how a woman could realistically make a decision regarding primary treatment if she didn't know whether she had the disease. She also questioned whether there might be characteristics of breast cancer that made one form of treatment advantageous over another. Rose was passionate on this subject and, more important, she was right. The amazing thing to me about this whole episode is that a patient advocate, not a doctor, single-handedly changed the care for women with breast disease almost overnight, forever.

Early in my breast cancer career, I had the pleasure of meeting Rose Kushner. She and Wendy Schain, our director of psychosocial research at that time, were friends, and Rose came to California to help launch our new breast center. She, more than anyone else, had brought about major changes in health care for women. Not only did she greatly reduce the number of one-stage mastectomies, but she began an advocacy movement for women's health issues that addressed the whole woman. This movement broadened into a demand for increased funding for breast cancer research, providing results for many years to come.

Women with newly diagnosed breast cancer now have choices.

They also have resources to help them make choices. A number of books are helpful, and these are listed in Resources at the end of this book. Many centers have peer mentoring programs where compassionate women who have been through the journey are available to share their experiences and give advice. It is natural for you to feel overloaded with information as you go about the necessary educational process of gathering information in order to make the best decision for you. Remember, you do have time. You can also have treatment in steps without compromising outcome. You will need time to think and consider options before making decisions. For some women, the decisions come easy; for others it can be much more difficult. There is no norm.

Some women are sure they want a mastectomy. The decision may be related to the characteristics of the cancer, or may have to do with family history or future risk, or logistical issues. When Nancy Reagan was found to have a very early breast cancer during the time of her husband's presidency, she chose to have a simple mastectomy. This upset a number of breast cancer advocates, who felt she should have chosen breast conservation. They publicly criticized her, alleging that she was setting a "bad example" for other women. Nonsense! She made the treatment choice that was right for her. I don't know what her decision was based on, but it was her decision. Some of my patients choose or require mastectomy and do not want reconstruction. Of course, reconstruction can always be done at a later time. A number of women leave reconstruction as an option for a later date and never feel the need to proceed. However, the vast majority who go on to have breast reconstruction are pleased with it and have no regrets.

We've come a long way from the days when there were no options other than mastectomy. But breast conservation is not the appropriate choice for all women. As advanced as we are, we know that there will be even more sophisticated surgical and reconstructive options to come. You must weigh all the risks, determine how the decision might impact your emotional, mental, spiritual, and physical self, and make a personal decision whether to keep or give up your breast(s).

❧ 8 ❧

Weighing the Risk

Risk is relative. For a new mother, a one percent increased chance to see that child reach kindergarten may be worth the greatest sacrifice. For the mother's mother, she would give that one percent for her daughter in a second, but not for herself in a lifetime.

—John Link

For many women a diagnosis of breast cancer is their worst nightmare. It is difficult to be rational and objective when you are blindsided with a diagnosis that could potentially end your life. This usually occurs at a time when you feel well and there is already enough on your plate. Suddenly all that seems unimportant. You are frightened and vulnerable in ways that you may never have experienced before. In this state of vulnerability you are probably willing to do anything that will help you survive. As frightened as you are, it is important for you to understand what you are up against. Knowledge is power and allows you to have control. The purpose of this chapter is to help you to make decisions based on knowledge, not fear alone. Remember, you have time to investigate and learn in order to make the best decisions for you. You do not have to master every nuance of breast cancer diagnosis and treatment. However, it is vitally important that you consciously pursue mastery sufficient to understand your choices as well as whom you should rely upon for expert advice.

How does invasive breast cancer begin? To be invasive, the cancer cells that reside on the surface of the milk duct must penetrate the *basement membrane*. This membrane separates the duct cells from the underlying fat tissue that contains blood and lymph vessels. When penetration takes place, there is the potential to spread, or metastasize, to distant places in the body. If this occurs and the cancer cells are not destroyed, the woman will ultimately die of breast cancer. This is not likely in breast cancer that is detected early. The factors that govern the ability of a cancer cell to penetrate a vessel are not clear, but the metastatic process is the subject of tremendous research. This chapter is about the risk of systemic spread and relapse as well as the potential interventions that apply. It is also about the complexity of this decision-making process in choosing those interventions.

A number of years ago a young woman came to me for a second opinion regarding her newly diagnosed breast cancer. She was thirty-two and she had a tiny, palpable lump on the surface of her left breast. She had just completed breast feeding of her six-month-old infant. The lump was a small cancer that was nine millimeters in size. It was removed and the first draining node was sampled using the sentinel node technique. The node showed no evidence of spread. In spite of her outlook being favorable, because of her young age and the way the cancer looked under the microscope, it was recommended that she undergo six months of chemotherapy. She came to me, accompanied by her mother, for my opinion regarding the need for chemotherapy. During the consultation, the mother revealed that she was feeling a small lump in her own breast and was concerned. I suggested that while she was at the center, she might want to see our breast radiologist for evaluation. She agreed, and unfortunately found she had almost the exact same type and size cancer as her daughter. Over the next several weeks both mother and daughter weighed the risks and benefits of undergoing chemotherapy. Each would receive approximately a

2 percent increased chance of being cured with the chemotherapy. After careful consideration the daughter decided that she wanted the chemotherapy, not only for herself but for the sake of her infant daughter. The mother, on the other hand, declined the chemo. At sixty-seven she did not want to trade present quality of life for a small increased chance of cure. She wanted to be at her full capacity to help her daughter through her battle with her cancer. To me this was a graphic example of the complexity of decision making about undergoing adjuvant systemic therapy. It is not only about the cancer itself; it is also about the person who has the cancer and her present life situation. Both women heard and processed the same information and then made different decisions that allowed them to proceed with their lives. It is now five years since I met the mother and daughter, and thankfully both are doing well.

My purpose here is not to describe in detail the latest adjuvant systemic treatments. Rather, I want to present the principles of the risks and benefits of systemic treatments to prevent relapse, since this book is about the empowerment that comes from taking charge and making decisions that are right for the individual woman. Information about the latest therapies will be available from your treating doctors and the Internet. In *The Breast Cancer Survival Manual* I have a chapter dedicated to the latest systemic therapies, and I also update women on our website, www.breastlink.org. The site is completely supported by private donors and receives no money or support from the pharmaceutical industry. Our intent is to provide the most current and accurate information possible without the influence of companies interested in selling their products.

As I have repeatedly emphasized, each woman's breast cancer is as unique as she is. Despite this uniqueness, I believe we will find similarities among various types of breast cancer that have common gene mutations. There is evidence that once a cancer develops, it is often genetically unstable. With further cell division, genes may mutate even more, causing the cancer to become more malignant. This probably explains why small, early, mammographically detected cancers are often low to intermediate grade on the scale we use to rate the aggressiveness of breast cancers, known as the Modified Bloom Richardson scale (MBR). (See *The Breast Cancer Survival Manual* for more information on this.)

As the cancer grows, mutations occur, with a greater potential for increased numbers of "outlaw" cells. Thus within the same breast cancer, there may be a number of different cell types. We call this intratumor heterogeneity, which refers to the variation within the tumor itself. As the cancer enlarges, it tends to grow faster, as the more rapidly growing cell lines take over. Unlike "normal" cells, which have a determinate cell life, a tumor cell fails to die. This process has treatment implications and may explain why only a percentage of cancer cells are hormone receptor positive (ER+). Intratumor heterogeneity also explains one of the theoretical benefits of combining different treatment modalities; for example, chemotherapy with hormonal therapy and, in the future, even gene therapy.

The Decision for Systemic Treatment

Unfortunately, we do not currently have a method to determine if cancer cells have escaped into the system. Presently we predict tumor behavior using models that include tumor size, lymphatic involvement, histologic grade, and gene abnormalities. We have not yet developed a highly accurate test to identify women with micrometastatic disease at the time of diagnosis. By micrometastatic, I am referring to single cells that have potentially escaped into the system. We must base treatment decisions on statistical probabilities. This means that at times we will use toxic therapies to treat women who are cured with local therapy alone and do not need adjuvant systemic

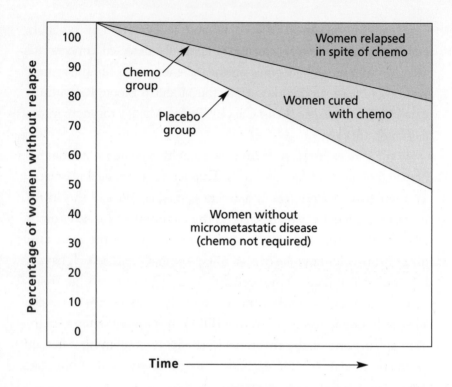

FIGURE 8.1
Results of a trial conducted in the 1970s

therapy. Unfortunately, some women with micrometastatic disease will still develop systemic spread despite adjunctive treatment. Figure 8.1 demonstrates this in graphic form.

This graph represents a group of women with invasive breast cancer at risk for micrometastatic spread treated with chemotherapy versus a placebo (the trial was conducted in the late 1970s). The vertical axis represents the percentage of women that are disease-free; the horizontal axis is time in years. The upper descending line represents the chemotherapy-treated women and the lower line the women receiving placebos. The area at the top of the figure indicates the women who relapse despite the therapy. The bottom area represents the group for whom therapy was not needed because these women did not have micrometastatic disease. The only women benefiting from the chemotherapy is the group in between. The large percentage of women, who are represented on this graph below the lowest line, do not have micrometastatic disease. If we had an accurate test to identify this group who are cured with local control alone, we could spare these women the unnecessary treatment and toxicity.

We also need a test to predict which women will relapse in spite of state-of-the-art therapy. In these cases, we learn at the time of relapse that the treatment was insufficient—whereas if we had this knowledge up front, a different approach could be taken to prevent relapse. Forced to choose between treatment and no treatment, we usually treat if the calculated risk of systemic recurrence is greater than 10 percent. When a patient recurs, in spite of systemic treatment, it usually happens because the tumor is resistant to the treatment agents chosen. We suspect there is a genetic basis for some types of drug resistance.

The best opportunity to cure a women with micrometastatic disease is before it is detectable by any of our present technologies. Once disease surfaces in the bones or lungs, the cancer is treatable, but not curable. The "time window" to treat and cure is when the burden of cells is at minimum. It would be helpful to treat only when the cancer surfaces in a relapse; but unfortunately, as we presently understand breast cancer, it is already too late to cure at this point.

Cancer cells may escape and migrate to a location distant from the original tumor. The presence alone of circulating cells in the body at the time of surgery does not mean that a woman will necessarily develop metastatic disease. The migrating cells must have the ability to survive and grow at a distant site—to establish blood supply. Many women are concerned that surgery or a needle biopsy might potentially spread cells into the system. There is evidence that even if this could happen, the cells will not establish themselves without the ability to recruit and stimulate blood vessel formation.

Tests are being developed that will allow us to measure tumor cell activity in the body more accurately at an earlier stage. Newer tests on single cells using antibodies that are labeled with radioactive tracers look promising in clinical trials in Europe. German scientists have been at the forefront in this research, and others are attempting to confirm their successful reports. What they do is take a bone marrow sample at the time of the original breast cancer surgery and then expose those cells to an antibodies cocktail that reacts to the presence of epithelial cells. Epithelial cells generate all the body's glandular and covering tissues. Theoretically, there are no epithelial cells in bone marrow. Breast cancer originates from a glandular epithelial cell. Therefore, a bone marrow sample that contains breast cancer will stain positive for this cocktail of antibodies. The test is very sensitive and can highlight one cell in a million bone marrow cells. If there are breast cancer cells in the bone marrow, we can assume that some breast cancer cells have escaped, but it is not clear whether these cells will actually take hold and form metastatic tumors. It is also not clear, as of this writing, whether the absence of breast cancer cells in the bone marrow reliably tells us that no breast cancer cells have escaped anywhere in the body. Yet, the bone marrow is certainly a good place to look. The marrow itself is like a vast net for the bloodstream and is thus commonly the site of the first sign of relapse in a majority of women.

While oncologists wait for this research to mature, they use other tumor characteristics to predict micrometastatic disease. Probably the most important of these predictors is lymphatic involvement—either by spread to the draining lymph nodes or by invasion of lymph vessels around the cancer itself. If the cancer has what it takes to penetrate a lymph vessel, then it makes sense that it can do the same to a small blood vessel. Indeed, many studies show that lymphatic spread has a strong association with relapse at a distant site. A correlation to the extent of spread to the lymphatics is that the more lymph nodes involved, the increased likelihood of a relapse.

Many women ask if the process of having a needle biopsy causes the spread of tumor cells. I need to make a distinction here. There is a difference between a cancer's ability to penetrate a lymph vessel and spread to the first draining (or sentinel) node and cancer cells being disrupted by a needle biopsy and picked up by the lymph system (which bathes all cells) and carried to the sentinel node. We are beginning to see many cases of the latter with the aggressive use of needle biopsies to diagnose early breast cancer. We do not think this iatrogenic (doctor-caused) spread is predictive of spread into the bloodstream and eventual relapse. In fact, after a diagnostic needle biopsy, a significant number of women with pure ductal cancer in situ (DCIS) will have a microscopic cluster of cells in the sentinel node. This particular form of breast cancer has no invasive ability; therefore, we know with certainty that the cells discovered in the lymph nodes are a result of the biopsy process. This occurs without any known negative consequence.

Cancer Spread Factors

Size of the primary cancer, or *tumor volume*, seems to be another critical factor in predicting systemic spread. As stated earlier, this is complicated by the tendency of cancers to be of a higher malignant grade as they grow larger, and indeed this may be more of a critical factor than the actual size of the invasive cancer. Swedish physician Laszlo Tabar has the largest database of small mammographically detected cancers. He has followed these women over twenty years and found that if the cancer is ten millimeters or less, regardless of malignant grade, the twenty-year disease-free survival is in excess of 95 percent. However, the size of tumor alone is not always sufficient to indicate definitively malignant potential. A woman with a tumor under twenty millimeters and of low malignant grade has an equally good twenty-year survival rate.

Breast cancers that are associated with certain altered genes tend to be more aggressive and spread earlier. We routinely look at two genes in particular: P53 and Her-2. The normal P53 gene helps repair DNA mishaps and keeps a cell from dividing until the critical DNA disruption has been repaired. When cancer cells have abnormal P53 (P53-positive), they are of higher grade and tend to grow faster. It is possible that the defective P53 gene has allowed the mutated cell to divide without repair.

The second gene we look at in breast cancer is Her-2/neu oncogene. I will go into more detail about this gene later, in chapter 10, where I discuss Herceptin, an antibody against Her-2 given intravenously. Cancers that overexpress, or make too much, Her-2 are more aggressive and spread sooner. With the current emphasis on gene research, we will likely discover other genetic abnormalities that will help us understand the nature of different types of breast cancer.

Cells that spread must have the ability to survive away from the primary tumor that produced them. They must divide and obtain nutrition. These malignant cells often produce factors that recruit blood vessels to provide the necessary nutrients and growth substances. Some of these so-called angiogenesis factors have been identified, and antibodies have been produced against them. A number of antiangiogenic drugs are currently in clinical trials. It is our hope that without the angiogenesis factors, cancer cells will not be able to grow.

Cancer cells definitely require external factors in order to survive and thrive. An example of an external factor is estrogen. More than half of all breast cancers have receptors for estrogen on their cell surfaces, meaning that these cells require estrogen in order to grow and divide. If the estrogen supply is interrupted, the cell may go into *apoptosis*, a programmed death cycle also called "cell suicide." Lacking enough estrogen, cells may be able to adapt and make more receptors on their surfaces. With the increased number of receptors, these cells may be able to trap tiny amounts of estrogen and survive. We know that besides the ovaries, other tissues such as fat and the adrenal gland can make estrogen by using an enzyme known as aromatase. A new class of drugs called aromatase inhibitors blocks this enzyme and has great potential to help women with estrogen-dependent breast cancer. Knowing whether your particular cancer is estrogen dependent is important for planning the kind of treatment you will need. Your surgeon or oncologist should take all the information about your cancer and provide an assessment based upon a statistical analysis of thousands of women in a similar situation and the percentage of those who remained disease-free over time.

No one can predict with absolute accuracy what will happen to you. I see women with highly malignant tumors and multiple positive lymph nodes who appear to be cured twenty years after initial treatment. Rarely, I will see a woman with a tiny node-negative cancer that ends up relapsing. The point is that you are not a statistic. You will need to take the information about your particular cancer and decide if you will need or accept adjuvant systemic therapy. In order to do this, you will need an honest explanation of the potential side effects of the treatment. Side effects are usually more acceptable if they are both temporary and reversible. Fortunately, most of the side effects that women experience from breast cancer adjuvant therapy are temporary and reversible. Once you understand the potential for increased cure, weighed against the time and toxicity of the treatment, you must decide if it is worth doing. As in the cases of the mother and daughter I described earlier in this chapter, other factors also enter into this decision-making process—such as age, underlying physical and mental health, and intuition—the inner feeling that you need to do it or not.

Systemic therapy penetrates the entire body regardless of where a cell has migrated. There are three classes of therapy that qualify to do this. I will briefly discuss each class, but remember, these areas are changing so rapidly that I will not make recommendations regarding optimal therapy. What I will do is state some principles and predict where we are heading with current research.

Hormonal Therapy

⬤ Breast cancer may be responsive to a number of hormonal interventions. Oncologists have access to a number of hormonal treatments that can potentially eradicate estrogen-sensitive cancer, which include SERMs (selective estrogen receptor modulators) like tamoxifen and toremifene; LHRH (luteinizing hormone-releasing hormone) agonists like Lupron and Zoladex; and aromatase inhibitors like anastrozole (Arimidex), and letrozole (Femara). Recent discoveries have given us a host of new agents that have replaced older treatments including testosterone, progesterone, and removal of the adrenal glands. We can predict if a cancer will respond to some type of hormone therapy by analyzing the cancer for estrogen and progesterone receptors. Many years ago, doctors observed rare cases of women with far-advanced breast cancer that spontaneously regressed when they went through "the change," or what we now call menopause. It was also observed over a hundred years ago that young women with far-advanced breast cancer would often go into remission if their ovaries were removed. These were the first clues that breast cancer is influenced by estrogen.

Today we have made progress, but there is still much to learn about estrogen's influence on breast cancer, an area that is receiving much attention by researchers. New hormonal therapy is targeted to the cancer, but there are side effects to estrogen-sensitive organs such as the vagina and the uterus. In premenopausal women, estrogen blockage or depletion may lead to hot flashes, vaginal lining dryness and thinning, mood lability, and calcium loss. We have developed a number of interventions that can minimize these effects and help women maintain their quality of life.

Ovarian ablation, or shutting down the ovaries' estrogen production, is the subject of renewed research interest. There are three ways to do this: surgical removal of the ovaries; hormonal agents that

reduce estrogen production; or cytotoxic agents that bring on menopause in young breast cancer patients.

Many oncologists are enamored of cytotoxic chemotherapy drugs.
This is due, first, to the dramatic responses they observed during their
training in treating leukemia, lymphoma, and testicular cancer. Second, chemotherapy administration is much more profitable financially
than an orally administered hormone pill. Consequently, oncologists
often bypass hormone therapy in favor of chemotherapy, usually to
the detriment of the patient.

Interestingly, part of the beneficial effects of cytotoxic chemotherapy may actually be hormonal. When young women with hormone
receptor–positive breast cancer are given chemo, one of the major
side effects is suppression of hormone production in the ovaries.
Those women who stop menstruating for six months or more have a
better chance of surviving than those who do not.

In my opinion, chemotherapy plays a minor role compared to hormonal therapy in the treatment of hormone receptor–positive breast
cancer. Adding chemotherapy to hormones provides a small statistical
advantage, as demonstrated by large randomized studies such as one
by the National Surgical Adjuvant Breast and Bowel Project's B20
study, which added two different types of combination chemotherapy
to the anti-estrogen tamoxifen in women with node-negative breast
cancer. We knew from a previous clinical trial, the B14 study, that
tamoxifen gave a significant survival advantage over placebo in this
group of women. The B20 study answered the next question, which
was whether, by adding chemo to the tamoxifen, there could be further improvement. The B20 data demonstrated that there indeed was
a small advantage to adding chemo—in the range of 2 to 4 percent.
The reason for this improvement with chemo may be that some of the
cancer cells will ultimately mutate and develop resistance to the hormone. The chemo would then be a backup defense. Another explanation, in premenopausal women, might be that the benefit of chemo

added to tamoxifen results from increased estrogen depletion by further suppressing the ovaries. We know that ovarian suppression alone in this group of women increases survival. The big question is whether this small increase in cure rate is worth the toxicity to the individual woman. This is a difficult question, and each woman needs to be educated to the risk and benefits and then decide for herself.

The various classes of hormone therapies are listed in the box below. In some cases, therapy may involve combining two different approaches to ovarian suppression—for example, combining the pituitary hormone LHRH agonist with a SERM or an aromatase inhibitor. As you can see, there are varied approaches to achieving estrogen depletion, providing a powerful line of attack on estrogen-dependent breast cancer. (See also chapter 11 and 14.)

· HORMONAL THERAPIES ·

Ovarian Ablation: Ovarian functions of producing hormones stopped.

> **Surgical**—Removal of the ovaries
> **Chemical**—By suppressing pituitary hormone (FSH, LH) function that stimulates the ovaries to produce estrogen (e.g., Zoladex, Lupron)

Additive

SERMs (Selective Estrogen Receptor Modulator): Class of agents that enter estrogen receptors and either block or stimulate. In breast cancer cells that are hormone receptor–positive, SERMs may cause apoptosis (cell death).

> **Tamoxifen** (Nolvadex)—Over twenty years in clinical use
> **Toremifene** (Fareston)—Approved for metastatic disease; may have less uterine stimulation
> **Raloxifene** (Evista)—Being tested as a prevention agent; approved for osteoporosis

Pure Anti-estrogen (Faslodex)—Known as an estrogen receptor down regulator, this monthly injection destroys the estrogen membrane receptors and puts the cell into its "death cycle"

Progesterone—Relegated to use after tamoxifen or an aromatose inhibitor has failed

Testosterone—Used rarely because of side effects

Aromatase Inhibitors: Prevents estrogen production in nonovarian tissue

Anastrazole (Arimidex)

Letrozole (Femara)

Cytotoxic Chemotherapy

Cytotoxics work by interfering with cell division. Although these agents affect all dividing cells in the body, cancer cells are much more sensitive to these agents than are normal cells for several reasons. You may be surprised to learn that cancer cells are actually quite fragile. With the insult of chemotherapy, they quickly go into a cell death cycle. Normal cells tend to be hardier and have stem cells to replace them if they die. Stem cells are precursor cells that produce new cells when they are needed. Cancer cells are dividing more frequently than most other cells in the body, and when they die, there is no stem cell counterpart to replace them. Breast cancers that are of high grade are most sensitive to chemotherapy. Fortunately, the low-grade cancers are almost always hormone receptor–positive, which gives us another effective method of treatment.

We now have almost fifty years of experience with chemotherapy. Breast cancer, as a heterogeneous group of malignancies, tends to be more sensitive to chemo than other types of solid tumors, such as lung cancer or gastric cancer.

The classes of cytotoxic chemotherapy used in the current treatment of breast cancer in the adjunctive setting are listed in Table 8.2 (see also chapter 10).

TABLE 8.2

Classes of Chemotherapy

Class	Mechanism
Alkylators: Cyclophosphamide (Cytoxan) Cisplatinum (Cisplatin)	Drugs that affect DNA and interfere with cell division. Act somewhat like radiation.
Antimetabolites: Methotrexate Fluorouracil (5-FU) Capecitabine (Xeloda)	These are false building blocks that are incorporated into the DNA and RNA strands leading to faulty replication and apoptosis. Xeloda is an oral drug that requires intracellular enzymes, which tend to be high in breast cancer cells, to be activated. This makes Xeloda more specific in its anticancer activity.
Anthracyclines: Doxorubicin (Adriamycin) Epirubicin (Ellence)	Product of a fungus and a type of antibiotic. Very active in killing breast cancer cells, particularly Her-2–positive cells. Attaches to DNA strands and sends cell into death cycle.
Taxanes: Pacilitaxel (Taxol) Docetaxel (Taxotere)	Product of the yew tree. Very active in killing breast cancer. Included in most node-positive, estrogen-negative protocols. Synergistic (said of two drugs that enhance each other; effect is greater than the expected addition of the two) with Herceptin and capecitabine (Xeloda).

Mitotic Inhibitor: Vinrelobine (Navelbine)	Attaches to machinery that allows migration of the chromosomes in cell division. Not usually part of most regimens, but may be soon because of its low toxicity and non-cross resistance (that is, the cancer cells that have resisted other types of chemo will respond to this class).

The chemotherapy agents tend to be used in combination, either given at the same time or given sequentially one after another. The purpose of using multiple drug regimens is to obtain synergy—to get a one-two punch. One drug may work only partially, but with a follow-up agent, the combination may be far more effective. The other reason for combining active drugs is that a few cancer cells may have mutated and developed resistance to the first drug but can be killed by the second agent at a time when their number is small.

There are dozens of different chemotherapy agents, but only a handful are used to treat newly diagnosed breast cancer. Many others have been tested in situations of more advanced disease without any advantage evidenced over those listed above.

The downside of chemotherapeutic drugs is that they are toxic—cell poisons—and there are side effects that vary in severity, depending on the individual woman. There has been tremendous progress in controlling most of the side effects from chemotherapy. Nausea and vomiting were major problems. They not only caused misery but worsened the situation by leading to dehydration. This further concentrated the chemotherapy and its by-products, which prolonged the nausea and vomiting. Fortunately, medications were developed that effectively address the chemical depletion that causes the severe nausea and vomiting associated with chemotherapy.

I emphasize the need to be well hydrated during the first seventy-two hours following chemotherapy administration. We have found that it is beneficial to have women receive intravenous hydration on either day two or three following chemotherapy, with day one being the day of administration. In spite of adequate oral fluid intake, our patients seem to do much better with the intravenous fluids for reasons that are unclear. I suspect that chemo may temporarily decrease absorption of fluids in the small bowel and other organs which can affect a woman's overall feeling of well-being. We need to do a study to confirm this, because there is certainly expense and inconvenience bringing a woman back into the clinic to be intravenously hydrated.

The major risk from chemotherapy is a temporary lowering of the white blood count, which puts a woman at increased risk of bacterial infection. This is potentially serious if the infection goes untreated, and can be life-threatening. It is the most critical reaction we monitor. Beginning at day seven to ten after administration of the chemo, the white cell count begins to fall. The lowest point is what we call the nadir count, and it usually occurs between day seven and day fourteen. Monitoring the first nadir count will usually allow us to determine how sensitive a woman's bone marrow function is to chemotherapy, as reflected in her white and red blood cell counts. We now have the ability to stimulate the bone marrow to produce white and red blood cells using special growth factors. One such agent, known as filgrastim (Neupogen), allows us to give full dosages of chemotherapy without delaying the scheduled next dose due to low white cell counts. Once the maximum benefit of a particular chemotherapy has been achieved, it appears beneficial to give a different drug to kill any surviving cells that might have developed resistance through some type of mutation or adaptation.

When do we know if enough is enough? Most of our knowledge comes from clinical trials. The current thinking is that when the systemic involvement is likely to be low—for example, in women with small, node-negative tumors—then four cycles using two or three active drugs, given every two to three weeks, are adequate. When the micrometastatic burden is likely to be higher (women with larger, aggressive tumors and/or involved lymph nodes), then more than four cycles should be given. The problem is that we have no tests that will tell us whether we are accomplishing anything. The microscopic cancer cells we are treating fall below the threshold of our best measuring techniques at this time. In other words, we are making an educated guess about the probability of micrometastasis and then about the amounts of drugs to eradicate the potential cells.

There is no question that cytotoxic chemotherapy is effective in eradicating certain subsets of breast cancer. Until we have another approach, we are stuck using chemo with all its unpleasant side effects. However, there is hope for new approaches as we discover the genetic basis for the various subsets of breast cancer.

New Proteins

With the introduction of the antibody Herceptin to the Her-2 receptor, we now have a whole new class of anticancer medications. In the future, we will have other proteins like Herceptin that inhibit angiogenesis or other drugs that can instruct a cell to go into apoptosis (cell death). Other proteins will be able to convert cancer cells back to their normal precursors. Presently, Herceptin has been FDA-approved to treat advanced breast cancer and is being tested in the adjuvant setting for women who have early breast cancers that overexpress Her-2 receptors on their cell membranes. This accounts for approximately 30 percent of women with newly diagnosed breast cancer. Antiangiogenesis agents are presently being tested in advanced breast cancer. Recently a medication, clodronate, which inhibits bone resorption, was tested in Europe in women with breast cancer. Preliminary results show a substantial reduction in the relapse rate in the women receiving this drug. Several ongoing clinical trials are attempting to replicate these results.

As scientists begin to understand the genetic events responsible for malignant transformation, targeted proteins can be engineered to reverse the process, prevent formation of cancer-feeding blood vessels, and prevent the growth of cancer cells. Until these are proven treatments, you may have the opportunity to participate in clinical research to test new anticancer medications.

To treat or not to treat is the critical question. We physicians need an accurate test to tell us if cells have escaped that can survive and cause metastatic disease and death. We also need a mechanism to determine if the treatment is or will be effective. Until we have these two predictive tests, we are recommending treatment based on statistics and probabilities. You are not a statistic. The best approach we have is to take all the information about your cancer and then present to you any interventions that can potentially improve both the quality and the quantity of your life. We also must weigh this against potential ill effects that you might experience. You need to be aware that as objective as your physicians try to be, they have their own issues that may prevent complete objectivity. Clearly the matter requires time and consideration.

∝ 9 ∝

The New Era: Genetics and Breast Cancer

Do not go where the path may lead, go instead where there
is no path and leave a trail.

—Ralph Waldo Emerson

In order to effectively advocate for yourself, it is vitally important to
have a rudimentary understanding of how breast cancer develops.
Increasingly, treatments are available that attempt to address the
genetic errors that contribute, in significant part, to the development
of a breast cancer. The blueprint of our physical being is contained in
forty-six chromosomes, the genetic information carrying units that
reside in each and every one of our cells. Our DNA code is fairly pure
when we are born, but certain cells can change as we age, in response
to various stimuli. I often hear patients diagnosed with breast cancer
comment that they have "bad genes." While it may be true that some
patients have inherited an increased genetic risk for certain diseases,
the truth is that we are at the pinnacle of evolution and our genes had
to be pretty darn good for us to be here.

After birth, cells can change or mutate, and these defects can lead to
diseases such as cancer. The cells that are prone to these mutations are
those that are exposed to our environment and that undergo stimulation and repeated division. These mutations occur by chance or are

secondary to environmental factors. A majority of these mutations are inconsequential, or silent, and have no "phenotypic," or physical, manifestation. A few, however, may lead to disease. Cancer is a disease that is caused by mutations in our DNA code. A few of us are more susceptible to cancer because we are born with an alteration of DNA that makes a cancer more likely to occur. About 10 percent of women who develop breast cancer have inherited changes in their DNA that place them at greater risk of getting breast cancer. Two genes, BRCA1 and BRCA2, have been shown to be responsible for a majority of these hereditary types of breast cancer. These genetic mutations are expressed in a woman's eggs or a man's sperm and, therefore, have the potential to be donated to offspring. The other 90 percent of women who develop breast cancer do so over the course of their lifetime. In these women, an alteration in the genetic code of a breast glandular cell results in the cell becoming cancerous. From that point on, the defect is passed to all new cells of the same type. It is important to understand that these acquired mutations cannot be passed on to children because these mutations do not involve the germ cells, that is, the egg or sperm. Therefore, the vast majority of breast cancers cannot be passed from a woman to her daughter (or son).

Mutated Genes

How does an altered section of DNA lead to a breast cancer? In the case of most breast cancers, we believe it requires several related alterations. To understand the process, you need to know some basic facts about the human genome. The *genome* is the DNA blueprint responsible for all the characteristics of your physical being: the shape of your face, the color of your eyes, your innate intelligence, your coordination, your immunity, and so on. Much of the information in the nucleus, or core, of a given cell is not used, but is kept in storage. A brain cell has the same genetic material as a breast cell, but is using only the brain part of the code; the rest of the cell's DNA is dormant. The overall master plan, so to speak, is dictated early during fetal life when cells, under the influence of various biological factors, become differentiated to have particular functions.

The scientists of the world have devoted tremendous effort, resources, and collaboration in the exploration of human genetics. The Human Genome Project is the foremost example of a multinational endeavor to map the complete human genetic blueprint. With a "rough draft" of the genome completed in June of 2000, we have begun to understand more fully what is genetically normal and what is not. The next steps will include determining the function of each gene and identifying the nature of the alterations in the gene sequencing that lead to the malfunction that is significant in the development of a disease process. This knowledge will affect treatment directly. A logical extension of this research will be advances in gene therapy that will restore the critically altered cell to its normal state. (An example of this is discussed in chapter 10, where we look at the development of Herceptin.) This new, genetic approach to disease, with increased dialogue among scientists, allows for rapid progress.

How do altered or mutated genes lead to the development of a breast cancer? The DNA template allows for the laying down of a messenger template. The messenger template determines the sequence or arrangement of the amino acids that form the proteins which are the directors of the body's activity. These proteins function as structural units of the body—antibodies, hormones, etc. There are proteins that act as messengers that tell a cell to divide (to start the cell cycle) or that instruct a cell to die and go into apoptosis (cell death). A number of mutations can, theoretically, lead to a breast cell becoming cancerous. In every case an abnormal protein is produced or a protective protein that prevents a cell from getting out of control is absent.

For example, in precancerous conditions of the breast, what we call hyperplasia, cells begin to divide too frequently. The stimulus for this seems to be hormonal influence; estrogen plays the key role and there may be no genetic abnormality at this stage. But with the cells proliferating too rapidly, they are vulnerable to mutations. When a mutation occurs, the cell becomes more abnormal with enlargement of its nucleus. The phrase that describes the altered appearance of the cell under the microscope is *atypical hyperplasia*. The cell is now recognizable under the microscope as precancerous. As the cell keeps dividing, it loses its ability to go into apoptosis, its natural programmed death. This loss of apoptosis is passed on to its progeny, and cells begin to accumulate and amass within the duct. This stage is termed *in situ* cancer because the cells are localized to the duct and have not penetrated beneath the duct lining cells into the underlying *stromal tissue*. In order for the abnormal breast cells to penetrate the lining, a genetic event is required that allows the cell to disrupt the natural barrier called the *basement membrane*. This involves enzymes that can dissolve or "drill" into the space beneath. In order to continue, the small collection of cells accumulating under the basement membrane must have nourishment. The next step is the stimulation to form new blood vessels, a process known as *angiogenesis*, which requires another genomic event.

Scientists have now identified some of these abnormally produced genes and the resultant proteins. As long as a newly developed cancer "stays put," and continues to grow only in the breast, it is curable. Some cancers, however, develop the ability to penetrate into lymph and blood vessels and spread to distant sites, the process we call *metastatization*. Once this has occurred, local treatment alone is not capable of curing or eradicating the cancer.

We are beginning to understand more about these precancerous phases of breast cell proliferation and some of the genetic changes that are responsible for them. I believe that the heterogeneous nature of breast cancer is due to the variety of genetic mishaps that can occur. Some breast cancers seem to have no premalignant phase: a critical mutation occurs and creates a highly malignant cell that immediately reels out of control—"born bad," so to speak. These cancers divide rapidly, and often hormones have no influence on them. As we begin to identify these different mutations in the DNA of the cancer cells, it is likely that many cancers will be found to have common defects. The mutated sequences of DNA that lead to the development of a cancer are called *oncogenes*. These give rise to an abnormal protein in the cell or cause a normal protein in the cell to be lost or silenced. A variety of techniques are being developed that will allow for rapid analysis of the abnormal genes in a cancer cell. For example, in a technique known as micro-array analysis, technicians compare a normal DNA sequence (plated out on a glass slide) and the DNA of a number of cancer cells, looking for differences. This will allow for genetic "fingerprinting" of the various types of breast cancers. The great hope is that having the genetic fingerprint of an individual patient's breast cancer will lead to gene and protein treatment that will correct or prevent the cancer process.

Types of Gene Mutations

Gene mutations fall into two major categories. The first mutation type leads to "gain of function." These genes code for stimulatory proteins that promote functions of growth, such as cell division, invasion, and angiogenesis. The second category is "loss of function" mutations. With this type of mutation there is loss of proteins that protect a cell. In normal, healthy cells the genes that code for proteins protect cells from going out of control. These proteins act as fail-safe mechanisms. If a normal cell mutates and begins the process of abnormal transformation, these proteins can stop cell division and even send the cell into apoptosis. With the loss of these protective genes and their proteins, cells are not "checked" and can go out of control, ultimately developing into a tumor. See the box on page 102.

· GENE MUTATIONS LEADING TO CANCER ·

I. *Gain of Function:*
These genes, known as oncogenes, lead to the production of proteins that promote growth, drug resistance, angiogenesis, penetration through basement membranes, etc.

- Epidermal Growth Factor (EGF) gene—involves the Her-1 through 4 genes that promote growth and proliferation.

- Bcl-2—encodes an oncoprotein that prevents apoptosis (programmed cell death).

- Cox 2 gene—promotes inflammatory reactions, but also promotes tumor proliferation.

- Multi-Drug Resistance (MDR1) gene—gives cancer cells resistance to various chemotherapies.

II. *Loss of Function:*
These genes, also known as tumor suppressor genes, mutate and lose their function, which is to protect a cell from developing harmful genetic mutations that lead to cancer.

- P53 gene—the most widely studied "loss of function" gene, associated with a number of human cancers, including breast cancer.

An example of a mutation that leads to "gain of function" would be a mutation and overproduction of one of the Epidermal Growth Factor (EGF) genes. There are a family of these genes, one being the Her-2/neu gene, which will be discussed in detail in chapter 10. Overproduction of these genes leads to growth of protein receptors on the cell membrane. These receptors attract small messenger proteins, or *ligands*, that stimulate the cell to divide, leading to the acceleration of the growth of the cancer. This accelerated cell division leads to further genetic mutation. Theoretically, this process could be reversed by interrupting the abnormal gene production or even interfering with the protein receptor's ability to receive stimuli. This type of approach makes much more sense than poisoning the cancer with drugs that affect all dividing cells in the body, including our healthy ones.

An example of a "loss of function" gene is the P53 gene. I call this the "watchdog gene," as its function is to protect the DNA in the cell. When a critical mutation occurs, the P53 gene activates and does not allow the cell to divide until the defect has been repaired. What happens, then, when a watchdog gene such as P53 fails in its function because it has mutated? The DNA within the cell is left unguarded, vulnerable to additional insult or mutation. It is estimated that 50 percent of human cancers have a mutated P53 gene. Tumors with abnormal P53 genes are more aggressive and are associated with a worse prognosis. These cells proliferate more rapidly and have a propensity to further mutate. Much research is being done to find ways to restore the normal function of the mutated P53 gene.

Treatments of the future will be oriented to restoring the normal function of these genes and, by so doing, stopping the cell mutations that lead to the development of a cancer. Other new therapies will involve the development of antibodies that will neutralize abnormal proteins that are produced by the mutated oncogenes. Amazingly, immune-impaired "nude" mice (along with the lack of immunity, these mice lack the ability to grow hair) are the ideal vehicle to test new biologic agents. Unable to reject the human tissue implanted in them, nude mice allow the researcher to readily measure the efficacy of the antibody.

This is just one of myriad technological improvements that facilitate the development of new treatments. Your awareness of these developments will arm you to be proactive, both now and in the future, in discussing your treatment options with your oncologist. For many of us, both patients and doctors, progress is not fast enough. Treatments that are state of the art today will be considered primitive in the future. That said, we are fortunate to have developed the level of sophistication we have in delivering these treatments, in minimizing side effects, and in increasing our expertise in maintaining patient comfort and well-being through treatment. Your task, in partnership with your physician, is to advocate to receive the best treatment available *now* and to take comfort in having done the very best you can.

❧ 10 ❧

The New Agents

Rational knowledge and rational activities constitute the major part of scientific research, but are not all there is to it. The rational part of research would, in fact, be useless if it were not complemented by the intuition that gives scientists new insights and makes them creative.

—Fritjof Capra

The developments in our understanding of the genetic underpinning of breast cancer have already led to some amazing new treatments. Because breast cancer is a heterogeneous, multifaceted disease, treatment methods will have to be equally diverse. The new understanding of breast cancer's fundamental genetic nature has resulted in a major shift in the nature of the research. Current trends in research are toward an approach based on underlying genetic alterations that are often responsible for the cancer itself.

Prior to this time in medical history, drugs evolved from what I call the "jungle floor." Substances harvested from nature were tested against a variety of cancers in the test tube. Many of the present chemotherapies were discovered using this methodology. These treatment agents were frequently the product of plants, fungi, or molds, hence the term "jungle floor." Adriamycin, for example, is the product of a mold. Taxol is the product of the yew tree. In the jungle floor model of drug development, huge numbers of substances are screened to find a single promising agent.

Once a promising agent is discovered, it is given to animals, usually nude mice, to study a variety of potential toxic effects to bone marrow, liver, and kidney. Breast cancer tumors can be implanted into mice that have had their immune systems altered in such a manner that they will not reject the human tumors. The new agent is then given to these mice and the response of the tumors monitored. If the new agent continues to appear effective, it is then given to larger animals; again, the researchers are looking for toxic effects.

If a jungle floor drug makes it this far, the next step is to apply to the Food and Drug Administration (FDA) for permission to do human testing. Human drug testing is done in three phases. Phase I is primarily a safety test. Small increments of the agent are given to human subjects with their permission. A whole battery of blood tests is performed after each dose, and the subjects are questioned regarding toxicity and side effects. If there is no major problem, then the dose is usually doubled, and then doubled again, until toxicity begins to appear. Most of the human subjects who volunteer for testing of a new cancer drug have advanced cancer. The response of the cancer to the new drug is monitored; however, in Phase I testing, the safety of the drug is the first concern.

Once the drug is proven to be safe, then it is given in sufficient dosages to hopefully achieve a response in the patient's cancer. This is Phase II testing, in which the scientist is looking for an objective shrinkage of the cancer. Volunteers for Phase II testing must have measurable tumors that can be monitored. Responses are defined by the degree of shrinkage of the measurable tumors. It is possible for a new agent to work on a certain subtype of breast cancer and not others. In the early part of Phase II testing, if a new drug gives a small percentage of positive responses, then larger trials will be conducted. The whole process is extremely expensive and time-consuming. If the drug continues to show promise and has tolerable toxicity, the pharmaceutical company developing the drug may apply for FDA approval to sell the drug for patients with advanced cancer. The company must show that the drug either improves the quality of or prolongs life.

Even after FDA approval, testing continues in comparative trials of the new drug against the standard drug treatments that exist at that time. These trials are known as Phase III trials. The whole process, from discovery on the jungle floor to FDA approval, can take years. Often a new and promising agent will make headlines long before it has been approved by the FDA for general use. However, it is important to be aware that these new drugs are in development and to ask your monitoring oncologist about how these new treatment modalities might affect your treatment or surveillance plan.

The new approach in drug development and research in breast cancer involves analyzing the individual cancer cell and looking at the difference between the cancer cell and its normal counterpart. Herceptin is an example of this new type of breast cancer research, which I believe will produce many more examples to follow. Herceptin is the first instance of developing a biological agent using rational research, not chance.

The Herceptin Story

The Herceptin story began in the late 1980s when researchers observed that certain ovarian and breast cancers exhibited an unusual protein on their cell surfaces not found on normal ovarian or breast glandular cells. Approximately 15 percent of breast cancers showed this abnormal protein. The cancers were more aggressive, with faster growth rates and poorer prognosis. Dennis Slamon, an oncologist and researcher at UCLA, was one of the first to document the presence of this abnormal protein. He observed an association between the increased amount of protein expressed on the cell surface and an increased growth rate of the cancer. Dr. Slamon then reasoned that this abnormal protein might be responsible for the aggressive manner in which tumors expressing the protein behaved. He and others found the responsible abnormal fragment of DNA. This fragment was called a variety of names, but ultimately became known as Her-2/neu. A normal cell has two copies of this gene sequence, but 15 percent of breast cancers, by some mechanism, make too many copies of this DNA sequence. As previously defined, a DNA sequence is termed an oncogene; the excess of the gene copies is called overexpression. Dr. Slamon and others further discovered that the abnormal cell surface protein was a growth factor receptor. The receptor theoretically picks up naturally occurring growth factors. Dr. Slamon hypothesized that perhaps an antibody could be made that would act specifically against the overexpressed, abnormal surface protein and thereby reverse this aspect of the malignant process.

Dr. Slamon formed an alliance with a premier genetic research corporation known as Genentech. In conjunction with the research and development scientists at Genentech, he pushed forward, through myriad obstacles, to develop the technology that would make this antibody a reality. Genentech then manufactured the antibody in sufficient amounts to begin clinical research. The next step was to test this substance, which would be called Herceptin, in women with breast cancer. Dr. Slamon applied for approval to test the substance through the appropriate FDA regulatory agencies and then applied through UCLA's Institutional Review Board to test the drug on women with terminal breast cancer that overproduced the Her-2/neu oncogene.

At the time, Dr. Slamon called me and described the new antibody. He asked if I might have patients with advanced Her-2-gene–overproducing breast cancer who would be interested in testing the new agent. He explained it was a Phase I trial and that he was concerned about determining the safety of the drug in human subjects. The protocol called for a small initial dose that would then be doubled each week thereafter. There was no indication except theoretic that the antibody might reverse a cancer.

At that time I was caring for a twenty-nine-year-old woman named Lynette Calderwood, who had widely metastatic breast cancer to her liver and was close to death. She was married to a fireman, Dave, and they had a three-year-old son, Travis, who was the love of their lives. Lynette had undergone every possible treatment in search of a remission and more time with her family. She realized that she was not going to see Travis grow up, but was willing to do anything to have more time with both him and Dave. After Dr. Slamon's call, I presented Lynette with the possibility of being part of this trial. She understood that she would be receiving a completely new and untested class of therapeutics. I explained that the chance of this helping her was very small. I also told her that it was an opportunity to further medical progress and maybe make a difference for women with breast cancer in the future.

Lynette did not hesitate. She wanted to try the new treatment. She went to UCLA to be part of the Herceptin program and was either the second or third human to receive the new treatment. It was very exciting and all the staff sensed that history was being made. At the time of her first Herceptin treatment, Lynette's liver was almost completely overtaken by the cancer and she was experiencing severe pain and profound weakness. To our surprise, she had no pain, nausea, or other side effects with the treatment. By the third treatment, which was still a very small dose, she was feeling better. I cautioned her to maintain a guarded optimism as it was too early in treatment to know if we had gotten an actual regression of the tumor. But Lynette continued to feel better. After eight treatments, Dr. Slamon ordered a repeat liver scan. The scan clearly demonstrated shrinkage of the spots on her liver. He called me immediately, ecstatic with this first evidence that several years of effort might really yield a breakthrough. Another patient was also responding. What had been a theoretical exercise, based upon an observation about the differences between the normal and abnormal genetic structure of a breast cancer cell, had led to the development of a viable new treatment for this particular type of breast cancer.

Lynette continued to improve. She was a vibrant, beautiful young woman with a supportive family. With increased enthusiasm, Dr. Slamon continued his quest to further test Herceptin. Genentech apparently was not convinced that there was enough evidence to make the financial investment necessary to produce sufficient Herceptin to do the next level of human testing. Dr. Slamon was undaunted and continued to put pressure on the company to push on. Lynette became the living embodiment of the potential of the drug and a "poster child" for the new discovery. Fortunately, Dr. Slamon was well connected to some important cancer research fund-raisers in Southern California. Through the Jonsson Comprehensive Cancer Center and the Revlon Breast Center, he met and gained the support of Ronald Perelman of Revlon, and Lilly Tartikoff, the dynamic wife of the late Brandon Tartikoff, who had been the head of NBC. With the money he and his supporters raised, he was able to reapproach Genentech. With its financial misgivings assuaged, Genentech agreed to gear up production of Herceptin. Much of this behind-the-scenes intrigue is chronicled in Robert Bazell's 1998 book, *Her-2*.

Of the twenty or so women with metastatic disease who entered the Phase I trial, only one was a long-term survivor. Several women, including Lynette, responded to treatment initially but then their disease progressed. Despite her widely metastatic disease, she'd lived a few extra months in which she cherished her family, saw Travis have his third Christmas, and contributed, along with many other courageous women, to the success of the fight to develop Herceptin. Based on the results seen with Lynette and several other women, Herceptin went into Phase II testing. By itself, it was proven to kill cancer cells effectively. It also enhanced the ability of standard chemotherapies to work in women with Her-2–positive cancer.

Correcting Genetic Mishaps

Herceptin's is the first of many stories to come, it is hoped, in which a genetic research observation leads to a scientific hypotheses, which leads to the testing of new compounds oriented to correcting genetic aberrations. Almost certainly we will discover that there are dozens of genetic mishaps that account for the numerous subtypes of breast cancer we treat. These mishaps translate into faulty protein synthesis; thus the key will be to identify the missing or abnormal protein and correct the situation, whether it means supplying a missing protein or blocking the activity of an abnormal one. We may actually develop the ability to repair the deranged genetic map. As with Herceptin, the pharmaceutical industry will play a pivotal role in this process. Recently I noticed an article in the business section of the newspaper announcing record earnings for Genentech. The major reason was profits from Herceptin.

In the pipeline are other new agents based on genetic abnormalities found in breast cancer. Some cancers produce proteins that stimulate new blood vessel development, or angiogenesis. One of these blood vessel–stimulating proteins is called vascular endothelial growth factor (VEGF). VEGF has been isolated and an antibody has been produced called anti-VEGF. It is in Phase I and II testing. There are also a number of gene and protein abnormalities being researched that will lead to new therapies. These therapies promise to be effective with little toxicity.

Since over half of breast cancers have hormone receptors on their cell membranes, there is tremendous interest in developing agents that can enter the cell at the hormone receptor and selectively disrupt the cell's proliferative mechanism. A whole new class of hormone treatment has recently been introduced, known as the *aromatase inhibitors*. These drugs, which are enzyme inhibitors, prevent estrogen production from nonovarian sources. They are highly beneficial in postmenopausal women with estrogen receptor–positive breast cancer. Another new agent, Faslodex (fulvestrant), actually destroys the estrogen receptor on the cancer cell surface, leading to cell death.

All of this new "smart research" is based on cell biology and genetics, rather than on a randomly discovered compound that indiscriminately poisons tumor cells and healthy cells. This new research is more cost-effective, and the time from discovery to treatment can be greatly accelerated.

Ultimately, however, this new system is dependent on you. Whether it is by being a willing participant in a clinical trial or contacting your senator or congressperson to advocate for research funding, you are essential to the development of new, less toxic, and more effective treatments. You do not have to be an expert in research to ask your doctor to be accountable to you concerning state-of-the-art treatment options—you just have to know that it is your right to ask.

Never Again

I have accepted fear as a part of life—specifically the fear of change. . . . I have gone ahead despite the pounding in the heart that says: turn back.

—Erica Jong

When it comes to cancer, there is one thing for sure—you never want to deal with it again. Once you have finished treatment, you need to move forward with your life, with a renewed awareness of your ability to choose *how* you will live. Think of Alice, who refused to start living until she was five years past her diagnosis, only to die, just after her fifth anniversary, from an unrelated cause (chapter 6). Once you have had breast cancer, your life is forever changed.

This chapter addresses the issues of follow-up care. For all breast cancer survivors, surveillance makes a difference. How you are "watched" will depend on the stage of the disease at diagnosis and on the tumor's response to the treatment. The truth is that 80 percent of women will be cured of their breast cancer—*cured*—never to return. However, because we cannot with 100 percent accuracy determine who will be cured and who will not, the question arises as to the manner in which survivors are followed.

Do women need myriad tests every few months? I do not believe so. With our present technology, if you relapse systemically, you can anticipate being in treatment on and off as the disease flares and subsides. This may change in the future as new treatments are developed that will allow us to cure a woman after a systemic relapse. The truth is that you and your doctors need to do everything you can at the time of your diagnosis, and then you need to resume life. Certainly you need periodic checkups on a regular basis. You need to be monitored for another breast cancer with mammograms and possibly diagnostic imaging. Your medical oncologist and breast radiologist should confer and come to a consensus about the frequency of mammographic screening. Because you have had one breast cancer, your risk of a second is slightly increased. Depending on your family history and other risk factors, your physician may want to do more than just an annual mammography. If you have a dense pattern on your mammogram, or if your first cancer was a lobular type, your doctor may suggest ultrasounds to alternate with your mammograms. Another surveillance method that is being looked at in high-risk women is MRI scanning of the breast. Although quite expensive, MRI appears to give information that conventional mammography cannot.

Once you have had breast cancer, a backache is never just a backache. Every ache or discomfort makes you ask, "Could this be the first sign of a recurrence?" It gets easier as time passes. Anniversaries come and go. That magical five-year survival mark is not quite as definitive of cure in breast cancer as it is in other types of cancer, but it is certainly a welcome milestone. Unfortunately, all women will carry the fear of recurrence to some degree for the rest of their lives. For most women, the "never again" feeling that arises in the course of treatment translates into an ongoing commitment to their quality of life.

Pursuing your quality of life becomes more complicated, though, once you have had breast cancer. Your awareness of the disease has increased a thousandfold. It seems a day does not go by without your seeing a magazine article or blurb on the evening news about the disease, or finding that an acquaintance has been diagnosed. Was this going on before you had breast cancer? Yes, but your awareness had not been raised to the same extent. Whether you share your experience with other women, particularly women who are newly diagnosed, will depend on how comfortable you are talking about the intimacies of your life. It certainly can be beneficial to hear the stories of other women who have made the journey. Each patient continues to make sense of her experience throughout her lifetime, and telling her very personal story may actually help her to process—emotionally, mentally, and spiritually—her breast cancer experience.

Many women ask what they can do to lower their risk of another breast cancer. I wish there was a magic formula to assure cure. There is no question that removing your remaining breast tissue substantially lowers your risk of another primary breast cancer, and some women certainly consider this. It makes sense for women who are BRCA1– or BRCA2–positive, in which the risk of another breast cancer is as high as 50 percent. Women with lobular carcinomas or neoplasia also have a substantially higher risk than the normal survivor for a second breast cancer, and many of these women consider bilateral mastectomies.

Hormone replacement therapy (HRT) increases your risk of a second cancer to a small degree. You need to balance the risk versus the benefits of being on HRT. An alternative to HRT may be one of the new SERM (selective estrogen receptor modulator) drugs. Raloxifene is the SERM approved for prevention of osteoporosis, and there are indications that it may reduce the incidence of future hormone receptor–positive breast cancers. The problem with Raloxifene is that it doesn't help much with vaginal dryness, loss of libido, or hot flashes. I am hopeful that in the near future we will have a better SERM that will do all the good things without increasing the risk of breast cancer.

What role do diet, exercise, and vitamin supplements have in preventing future breast cancer? Again, there is no definitive answer. I am certainly not opposed to a well-balanced, low-fat diet and vigorous exercise. Whether they help prevent breast cancer is not proven, though under study. There has also been a surge in research interest in naturally occurring, as compared to laboratory-made, compounds, and we are hopeful that many of these, or their clinically active parts, will be proven effective against many forms of cancer. We are not there yet.

A distressing perception among American women is that breast cancer is a leading cause of death. This is far from true. Slightly less than 4 percent of American women die of breast cancer and this number is shrinking. It *is* a leading cause of death of women between forty and fifty. This is because women at midlife are generally extremely healthy and at low risk of death from other cancers, cardiovascular disease, and AIDS. The leading cause of death of American women is far and away heart disease.

Among the protective factors against recurrence are radiation therapy and hormonal therapy. Radiation to a breast seems to protect the breast for about five to seven years, and then the risk returns to the level of the nonradiated breast. This makes sense, since we think it takes five to seven years for a small cancer of several dozen cells to reach the size at which it can be detected on a mammogram. The radiation not only destroys cancer cells that may have been left behind at the time of surgery but also eradicates tiny unrelated cancers in the affected breast.

Tamoxifen and other SERMs such as Raloxifene may also give some protection from future new breast cancers. This protection would appear to be only for estrogen receptor–positive cancers and would not help women who had hormone receptor–negative cancers. About 50 percent of breast cancers are hormone receptor–positive. The evidence of SERM protection from a second breast cancer comes from clinical trials using tamoxifen after surgery to prevent systemic relapse. Tamoxifen did reduce relapses, but there also appeared to be a reduction in new hormone receptor–positive cancers. This observation led to a prevention trial that tested tamoxifen against a placebo in women of moderately increased risk of breast cancer. Approximately

14,000 women entered the five-year study. It confirmed that tamoxifen reduced the number of hormone receptor–positive cancers but was associated with a slightly increased incidence of uterine cancers and venous thrombosis. We will probably never know if the tamoxifen group has a reduced death rate from breast cancer, since these cancers are usually the most detectable and treatable. For those women who develop hormone receptor–negative cancers, we need a strategy that will subvert these potentially lethal cancers, the "born bad" type, that enter the bloodstream early.

The first SERM prevention trial spawned a second trial, known as the STAR trial, that will compare tamoxifen to Raloxifene in women over age fifty. Raloxifene has the potential advantage of not increasing the risk of uterine cancer. In my opinion, neither drug is ideal for prevention. Both drugs have potential side effects and the expense is tremendous. A year's prescription is a thousand dollars or more, and the recommended length of time of administration is a minimum of three to five years. It is clear from the prevention trial that tamoxifen modestly reduces the development of hormone receptor–positive breast cancer. What is not clear is whether it reduces mortality. With this in mind, women should carefully weigh the potential benefit versus the potential side effects associated with this medication.

Unfortunately, you cannot prevent a second breast cancer. If you survive a first episode, which is highly likely, your chance of a second cancer is *slightly* increased in comparison to women who have never had breast cancer. The exception to this is if you are BRCA1– or BRCA2–positive or have lobular neoplasia. These variations increase your breast cancer risk to a degree that may cause you to consider surgical preventive strategies. Otherwise, you need to go on with your life and continue screening. "Never again" in terms of a second breast cancer can only be understood based upon the surveillance tools we have available at present. There will be new methods for breast cancer surveillance over time, and your oncologist should be able to apprise you of these in your regular follow-up visits.

The Mind Is a Powerful Thing

What Cancer Cannot Do

Cancer is so limited . . .
It cannot cripple love
It cannot shatter hope
It cannot corrode faith
It cannot destroy peace
It cannot kill friendship
It cannot suppress memories
It cannot silence courage
It cannot invade the soul
It cannot steal eternal life
It cannot conquer the spirit.

—Author unknown

Breast cancer is a cruel disease. Most women are blindsided by the diagnosis—they are in the middle of their lives, taking good care of themselves, when suddenly their lives are threatened. One day life is normal, and the next, it is upside down. Unlike heart disease or lung cancer, which can be caused by lifestyle, there are no definite known causes of breast cancer. It often strikes women who are, apparently, in the best of health. For most women, the diagnostic process proceeds something like this. The first sign is an abnormal mammogram or a lump that wasn't there last month. *You are frightened and concerned.* Next, there is a biopsy and the results return: malignant. *You are stunned.* The medical oncologist then outlines an advised course of treatment for you. He or she uses the words chemotherapy, lumpectomy, mastectomy, and radiation. *And it all feels unreal.* There are treatment decisions to be made, and in this state of shock and disbelief, you are expected to become educated and make decisions that will, along with the diagnosis, change your life forever. With these blows still echoing in your mind and heart, you *will* make decisions. For most women this is the fight of their lives—not just physically, but emotionally, mentally, and spiritually as well. Through numbness, despair, anguish, anger, and disbelief, a treatment plan will be pursued and begun. Balancing your emotional states while moving forward with treatment is an art. It requires a resilience which I see women develop with each step in treatment each day. There are no rules for how to do this—each woman must find her own way. There are, however, some commonalities in the experience, which may be helpful to understand.

Prior to their diagnosis most women make a basic assumption about their body—that it will not allow an illness or disease to develop without sending out strong distress signals. Then a breast cancer is diagnosed. There has been little history of distress—in most cases there was, in fact, no distress at all prior to discovering the lump. The awareness that a life-threatening illness has developed "under your nose" is astounding. Trust in the body is gone. The most fundamental sense of trust and safety has evaporated—in an instant.

To the extent that you have had unpredictable life experiences previously, you may have developed successful strategies for managing crisis. Even with the most sophisticated coping skills, this crisis is challenging. On the other hand, the experience of earlier life crises may simply have left you shell-shocked and made you more vigilant or watchful rather than more resilient. And it is resilience that you will need.

Fortunately there is a wealth of psychological research on resilience, learned optimism, and the reframing of painful experiences. One of the most powerful principles of crisis management, from a psychological perspective, is the ability to find an aspect of the traumatic experience that is meaningful to you.

Many years ago, I recommended radiation therapy to a patient who was a devout Christian. She was, interestingly, the wife of a physician and was deeply in conflict as she tried to reconcile her faith with the recommended treatment. She prayed many times each day and could envision what she described as "the light of Christ" healing her. However, she also felt that she would live with regret if she did not choose to complete the treatment as prescribed. She wrestled with this dilemma and returned to see me after she had started treatment. She told me that she had decided that she would focus on the radiation therapy as the outward manifestation of a process that was ongoing for her; radiation had become a representation of the light of Christ and was available to heal her. Not only did she complete her treatment, but she felt a real peace each day when she went in for treatment. In this way, this patient made the treatment truly her own, investing it with meaning that was personal and that gave her a sense of control.

Often we will hear a patient, seeking some meaning in this crisis, say: "I don't believe that I was somehow 'given' this cancer in order to learn something, but as long as it's here, I think I'll review how I'm living my life and see what I'd like to be different." Something has happened in each woman's physical, mental, and emotional environment as a whole that allowed a cancer to develop. Though we do not know what the critical alterations were, these patients find or define changes they wish to make that may, in fact, positively impact this environment. At a minimum, each woman has a sense of power in choosing areas for change in her life, as opposed to submitting to the changes necessitated by the cancer and its treatment. Beyond treatment, each woman will continue to decide whether or not she will assertively define the role cancer will play in her life or whether she will live her life in the shadow of the cancer experience. The commitment to changing or reaffirming meaningful areas of your life often helps to give you a new sense of security, not in the body per se, but in your own ability to take back control and to improve, in a lasting way, your quality of life.

Women who seem to have the most difficulty with the breast cancer crisis are those who have experienced a major trauma earlier in life. Often this earlier crisis has been suppressed or is unresolved. Most women will not see a connection between the overwhelming reaction they are experiencing with their breast cancer and these prior traumas. However, the body does not forget. In these moments of emotional upheaval, these women frequently feel flooded with a crippling sense of loss and a sense of doom that goes beyond even that which is experienced with a cancer diagnosis. In this situation, the breast cancer evokes a type of post-traumatic stress disorder that impairs concentration and decision making. These women are particularly vulnerable to depression and anxiety. Psychotherapy can be extremely helpful in this situation—the breast cancer may in fact provide the opportunity for these women to resolve issues of their previous, unresolved trauma.

During the period when a diagnosis of breast cancer is such a shock, many women can benefit from psychological support and counseling. Although women can and do "get through it," it is often beneficial to have assistance in managing this crisis. Many medical centers have psychotherapists and social workers who are available for women with newly diagnosed breast cancer. Depending on where you live, access to professional help may not be this easy, but with some effort you should be able to find a qualified counselor or therapist to help you through this.

Each newly diagnosed woman with breast cancer has a unique life experience and social support that she brings to her disease. Many women have partners—husbands or significant others—who will offer various degrees of support. While some partners seem to move forward with little difficulty, sometimes the amount of support partners can give is limited by their own distress. It is also simply not possible for "outsiders" to completely understand a major life crisis such as newly diagnosed breast cancer. Your priorities, your goals, and your attachments are not the same. Questions that no one can answer may haunt you. Could you have prevented it by being more vigilant? If you are more vigilant now, can you prevent a recurrence or another catastrophe in the future? Did you somehow contribute to the development of your cancer? These thoughts and questions are common and a critical part of the process of trying to understand how this cancer occurred. Ultimately, each woman will decide whether or not her thoughts will remain focused on unanswerable and anxiety-provoking questions, or whether she will move forward, with added clarity, in her pursuit of quality of life *now*.

The opportunities for transformation begin the moment you are diagnosed and will continue for the rest of your life. This transition from reactor to action taker may also involve a certain amount of stress, but it is the healthy stress of finding a more empowering way of being, through crisis. That said, you may have trouble sleeping and eating, both because of the crisis and because of the treatment. These changes may contribute to an actual imbalance in your brain chemistry, since the chemicals which regulate your mood and appetites are affected. Your family, although well-meaning, may add to your stress. Your physicians may take you off replacement hormones, resulting in intense hot flashes and other menopausal symptoms. Chemotherapy may put you into premature menopause or worsen existing menopausal symptoms. These biochemical stressors may result in depletion of a chemical called *serotonin*, which is a neurotransmitter that regulates circadian rhythms, waking and sleeping, as well as your appetite for food and sex. When serotonin is depleted, it can lead to depression and feelings of chronic despair as well as problems with sleeping, appetite, and decreased sexual desire. It is appropriate to have feelings of depression and despair with a diagnosis of breast cancer. Many women rally and address the problem and move on without much fuss. Others, devastated and overwhelmed, have difficulty in coping and decision making.

All women initially feel overwhelmed, but each of you has your own style of coping with stress and life's challenges. Breast cancer never comes at a good time, but for some it is worse than for others. As doctors, we are proactive in taking care of the physical issues: removing the tumor, ordering tests, prescribing medications to prevent relapse, etc. But we often fail to inquire what is really going on inside a person. Frankly, many physicians don't really want to know. The feelings associated with treatment may overwhelm their resources and cause physicians to feel powerless.

What many women need at this time is a physician who can bring his or her humanity, *his or her whole self*—feelings and all—to the situation. It is not that physicians don't care; it's that they are often not comfortable dealing with feelings. Or it may be that the energy required to do this is too great. It's the story of the busy surgeon who ends up performing a one-stage radical mastectomy on Mrs. Jones for what was thought to be a benign lump. At his first visit the next day to check his patient, he greets her and touches her hand. "The good news is that we got it early," he says. "I was able to remove all of the cancer." The bad news is obvious. He tells her that she is not the first woman to have this happen, and that the volunteers from "Reach to Recovery" or a similar support group will stop by in the next day or so. Then he quickly moves on to his next hospital patient. Physicians are educated to perform the tasks that are within their area of expertise and then to move on.

Support programs may help to provide you with a shared emotional experience and understanding as well as provide a forum to discuss all your concerns in a time-friendly format. Such programs are not a substitute for empathic doctors and staff. However, they are extremely potent resources for you, the patient. In our center, we have a peer-mentoring program called Breast Friends, which matches a survivor with a newly diagnosed patient. We try to match women based on similarities in treatment and life situation. It is extremely empowering for a newly diagnosed woman to meet and talk with a woman who has "been there" and is now back. I am convinced that these patient-to-patient interactions are worth hours of counseling and education.

Every oncology consultation should include a discussion of the patient's personal resources and support network. Our approach involves providing women, when appropriate and requested, the following resources:

1. Access to our support program, which involves individual counseling with a licensed social worker or psychotherapist, peer-mentoring, and several support groups.
2. Recommendations regarding diet and exercise.
3. Recommendations for alternative or complementary care, for example, acupuncture.
4. Assessment regarding the benefits of short-term use of psychotropic drugs for anxiety, insomnia, or depression.

We believe diet and exercise are important not only from a physical aspect but also psychologically. With the diagnosis and all that surrounds it, most women feel loss of control. Diet and exercise are areas that you can control. Taking back control over these aspects of your life, as well as of any other areas that feel significant, empowers you and helps you feel confident.

Exercise is also extremely important in developing and maintaining a general sense of well-being. One of the many beneficial effects of exercise is related to endorphin release and its impact upon brain chemistry, neurotransmitter levels, and mood. We know that regular, vigorous exercise increases natural endorphins, which give a sense of well-being and pleasure. Many women who were athletic prior to the diagnosis often feel discouraged that their active lifestyle did not protect them. Nevertheless, studies show that women who exercise regularly tend to cope and function at much higher levels than women who do not. We are even finding that exercise helps women overcome the fatigue that often accompanies chemotherapy and radiation. Many patients find gentle, nonaerobic exercise such as yoga extremely helpful and calming. Again, it always requires a balance between reclaiming physical strength and stamina and overstressing an already sorely taxed body.

Diet, exercise, and nutrition are helpful in reclaiming a sense of control over your body. However, the most powerful tool that you have in the fight to manage this crisis is your ability to think and feel. The breast cancer diagnosis is frequently so overwhelming that it leads to feeling stuck, unable to move, unable to think or choose to alter the outcome. Nevertheless, you *will* begin to move again, and when you do, it is important to remember that you have the final word with breast cancer—you will decide the place this disease will assume in your life, while in treatment and beyond.

ଊ 13 ๛

Faith, Healing, and Miracles

Faith in the gods or saints cures one, faith in little pills another, hypnotic suggestion a third, faith in a plain common doctor a fourth. . . . The faith with which we work . . . has its limitations [but] such as we find it, faith is the most precious commodity, without which we should be very badly off.

—William Osler

Webster's *New Dictionary* defines faith as the belief in the truth, value, or trustworthiness of someone or something. Each and every patient brings her own set of beliefs about the cause and healing of her breast cancer. When I ask patients "Do you have any ideas about what caused this cancer?" they more often than not have a specific belief about why they have this disease. Although traditional medicine is not yet able to affirm or deny these beliefs, we know that they are a powerful influence in the patient's ability to receive treatment and to pursue her "healing," not just her cure.

Belief about what leads to healing is in the realm of faith. Ultimately the extent to which the treatment path you pursue is right for you will be determined by the extent to which you have integrated it with the voice of your soul. We know from years of clinical trials that if a person believes in a particular treatment, it is much more likely to be successful than if the person has no "faith" in it. I truly believe that there is something about faith that promotes healing. I can't explain it in traditional scientific terms. The inability to quantify it, however, does not diminish its effectiveness.

About twenty years ago I met a young woman named Rosalyn L. Bruyere. I was introduced to Rosalyn through a mutual friend who wanted me to meet this very gifted "spiritual healer." I have always been open to new ideas and concepts, but this was a stretch for me. We met at a social gathering. She was in her early thirties and had bright sparkling eyes and red hair and a wonderful smile. I think I expected to meet a "witch" out of a Roald Dahl story, but she was delightful. It was clear from the outset that she was very intelligent. She had studied electrical engineering in college and had a somewhat normal life as a wife and young mother.

That evening, she described knowing that she was different even as a child, with an ability to "see things others could not." She said it was a little frightening and she was hesitant to tell others about her "gift," in that she was concerned about people thinking she was crazy or odd. So she resisted exploring this special ability. She seemed to know when people were sick, and if she touched them, she had the ability to ease pain and discomfort. It was only when Rosalyn's three-year-old son told his mother that he could see different colored lights around people's bodies that she felt the need to understand what he was experiencing in order to explain it to him. Her sons, Joe and Mark, both described seeing the same color fields, or "auras," that she had been seeing as long as she could remember.

Rosalyn began to explore her ability to interpret light and energy emitting from others. She sought information about the phenomenon in scientific literature, and she searched for others who had similar abilities. She began to study the works of the American Indian shamans as well as ancient healers of Egypt and Asia. In seeking to understand and to quantify her abilities, she developed a rare talent for moving between cultures, honoring the sacred traditions of each, and gathering information on their beliefs about healing. She has committed her life to teaching these practical tools for healing. I have learned much about this through my years of encounters with her. She is humble and reserved about her healing skills. In fact, she believes that the ability to heal resides in anyone who actively pursues his or her potential. I have never heard her boast, nor does she use her gift for personal fame or fortune.

I cannot see the lights that she sees around people nor understand their significance. When she puts her hands close to me, I can feel a strange electrical sensation on the surface of my body below her hands. The incredible thing is that she is able to diagnose illness in different areas of the body with her senses. Rosalyn's ability has been scientifically verified at the UCLA Laboratory of Applied Kinesiology with Professor Valerie Hunt in 1978 and as recently as 1994 at the Menninger Clinic's Center for Applied Psychophysiology in Topeka, Kansas, with Dr. Elmer Green. My patients who have seen her describe a significant relief of pain and improved ability to tolerate treatment after experiencing her "running energy" with them. While I do not know how she does this, I am convinced that the effect is real.

Rosalyn is a fascinating person and has a fascinating ability. To her credit, she has become one of the foremost healers in the world. Though she once had an extensive healing practice, she has given it up in order to pursue teaching and research. Presently she works with Dr. Andrew Weil and his program in integrative medicine at the University of Arizona, and three times a year she travels to the Kennedy Krieger Institute in Baltimore, Maryland, where she works on infants with neurological disorders.

What I have observed in my patients verifies the effectiveness of her approach to healing. I feel extremely fortunate to have met Rosalyn relatively early in my professional career. Knowing her has helped to remind me that there are many approaches to healing. I believe that Western medical education alienates the young physician from a richer approach to the healing process by encouraging him or her to discount that for which we do not have well-developed, scientifically tested explanations.

I have always felt that this limitation in medical training should be challenged, and for several years had the opportunity to do so in a course I taught to first-year medical school students at the University of Southern California. I invited Rosalyn to meet with the students I was teaching in a course called "Introduction to Clinical Medicine." Rosalyn is a superb teacher and she was wonderful with the students. She talked with them about what she did and she demonstrated "laying on of hands" and "running energy." Although they were as skeptical as six young medical students could be, they left with an appreciation that there is more to healing and medicine than was being taught in their curriculum. The administrators of the medical school heard of our meeting with Rosalyn and asked that I not bring her to the class again. They felt it was "too confusing" for the medical students this early in their careers. I had to laugh at this response. If the students' ability to keep an open mind and willingness to consider other paradigms of healing would have a harmful effect on their medical education, then it seemed to me that traditional medicine would eventually be doomed by its own near-sightedness.

Physicians are asked to ignore perspectives on healing that are not quantifiable by traditional methods. We are asked to sweep them under the mind's rug, asked to discount or invalidate what we cannot explain. The scientific method promotes our mechanical understanding of the body, its functions, and disease. However, no single method can address how disease develops within the complex relationship of mind, body, emotions, and soul, which characterizes our existence. Each healing discipline views medicine and treatment from a unique perspective. The tendency is to believe that the perspective in which you are trained is the only legitimate perspective. My hope was to stimulate young professionals early in their careers to remain open to that which they do not understand, both within their own discipline and across disciplines.

I also believe that cultivating an openness to our patients' beliefs about healing is an integral part of patient care. I am privileged to be the medical director of three breast centers in Southern California and have an opportunity, in this role, to challenge our staff to remain open to each woman's beliefs about her illness. We try to treat each woman as a unique individual, applying the best that science has to offer, tailored to her situation. With these goals in mind, we created a company retreat, which we called "The Culture of Healing." One of the speakers, Dr. O. Carl Simonton, wrote a revolutionary book over twenty years ago entitled *Getting Well Again*. At that time the book was extremely controversial. These were still the days when a one-step Halsted radical mastectomy was the recommended treatment for breast cancer. The very idea that you must treat the whole person, not just the tumor, was more than a decade away. At the time, Dr. Simonton was bold enough to suggest that through visualization and focused imagery a patient could impact his or her outcome in fighting a disease—in this case, cancer. As a radiation oncologist, he had observed that patients who took an active role in their care using visualization, guided imagery, and positive thoughts did better, lived longer, and expressed more satisfaction in their treatment and a greater sense of control. The academic community went crazy and the American Cancer Society called him a quack. His career as a traditional radiation oncologist was ruined. It is interesting that the tenets put forth by Dr. Simonton in the late seventies and early eighties are readily accepted today not only in medicine but in other areas as well. Sports and business psychologists, for example, preach the principles that positive imagery and visualization improve performance and affect outcome. Most of us dealing with cancer patients know that if patients feel consistently hopeless and helpless, it inhibits their ability to participate actively to achieve optimal care. That which empowers patients to actively participate in their care facilitates healing. If the treatment is done not only *to* the patient but *with* the patient, healing of body, mind, and spirit is more easily achieved.

At our retreat, Dr. Simonton shared these principles with us as they had evolved for him. He discussed psychologist Martin Seligman's research in "learned helplessness," which indicates that any individual who is unable to meaningfully impact her life in a consistent manner is likely to suffer from depression and an impaired ability to be proactive in her own care. Interestingly, these defeated and depressed patients also express a powerful belief, verified by their life experience, that their efforts do not count. These patients are less likely to eat well, have more physical pain, use more pain medication, and, I believe, die sooner in most cases. Dr. Simonton spoke to us about the potency of patients' beliefs and the manner in which these beliefs affect their attitudes and feelings about treatment, even their "will to live." He spoke with our staff about how to support individual patients who have not always felt effective in advocating for themselves. It was a wonderful experience for us to learn from Dr. Simonton. He is a gentle, thoughtful man of conviction and courage. He is committed to one purpose—to help patients feel that every part of them—body, mind, and spirit—has a powerful voice.

Over the years I have frequently observed that when patients would read Dr. Simonton's book, they felt empowered and less victimized. If patients become involved in their treatment and become partners with their physicians and caregivers, they are more positive and feel more in control. One of the undercurrents of criticism of Dr. Simonton's work was that if there were things the patient could do to *get well*, then maybe there were things the patient was doing that contributed to disease. The extension of this was that perhaps the patient caused his or her disease. It was not the result of something you thought or ate. Breast cancer is the sum total of many "hits," a variety of insults to the body that result in change at a cellular level. Regarding this, let me be absolutely clear—*you did not cause your breast cancer*.

However, I am frequently queried about the relationship between stress and cancer. On almost a daily basis, I am asked, "Dr. Link, do you think the terrible stress I've been under caused my cancer?" A number of years ago psychologist Lawrence LeShan posited a connection between stress and cancer. He actually went so far as to develop a life-stress scale. He listed stressful events such as a death in the family, divorce, marriage, or job change and gave each a score. Even positive events could add stress and thus were rated, too. Cancer patients could look back at the year prior to diagnosis and give themselves a score. These scores could be compared with those of a friend or brother who didn't have cancer. The conclusion was that many cancer patients had high scores in the year prior to their diagnosis. It was an interesting theory. The theory was predicated on the concept that stress weakens the immune system and the body's ability to fight off cancer. The problem with the theory is that most cancers are five years old before they are discovered. The truth is, life is stressful. What we want are more positive stressful events than negative ones: births, promotions, exciting new relationships, etc. This is called having a full life. Unfortunately, negative stressful events are inevitable. It is how we manage them that is important. Vital in stress management is the significance which we impute to a given event. Significance is determined by the interpretation of the stressor, the meaning attached to the stressor. Some patients, for example, feel that cancer is just the icing on the cake after a lifetime of unmanageable crises. Others, with similar histories of crises, see breast cancer as a life challenge, without reference to some ominous future.

I believe that how we interpret events is critical in the evolution of an event from a stressor to an oppressor. The chronic experience of oppression and powerlessness leads to depression and despair. Unresolved stress means that you are in a situation or a relationship that seems hopeless and unrelenting—in which there is no end in sight.

Loss of control seems to be the critical factor. A number of animal experiments demonstrate this. Animals put in situations where they lose control and receive intermittent negative stimuli lose weight, develop sores on their body surface, and die.

One of the many lessons inherent in the experience with breast cancer is the stimulus to take back control of your life. Chronic stressors such as a tyrannical boss, an abusive spouse, or a teenage child out of control may be more resolvable than they seem when compared to the stress of having cancer. Undoubtedly, one of the ultimate stressors in life is cancer. The Simonton book was so important because it offered a means of control to cancer patients receiving intermittent negative stimuli (radiation, chemotherapy, pain). Through the use of guided imagery, they could control, to some degree, what was happening to them. The visualizing patient was able to take powerful positive action against these stimuli and transform the experience.

Are Miracles Possible?

Do miracles occur? Absolutely. My definition of a miracle is an unexplained event that is positive and good and is very much desired or hoped for. As a scientist I cannot explain miracles. I see lots of them, though. Sometimes I am given credit for them as a physician, but in my heart I know that it happened in spite of me or my medicine. For those who believe in higher powers, miracles are easily explained. For those like me who struggle with faith, miracles are problematic. I know that I see miracles every day—in my patient Toni, for instance, diagnosed with advanced breast cancer, who decided that joy is her life's work. This lovely woman had always felt valued by her family and friends for her career choices. After her diagnosis it became clear to her that she felt emotionally and spiritually dead in her career. During treatment her husband died. In the midst of this tremendous grief, she continued to seek some meaning in her losses. She made the decision to eliminate from her life every aspect that was not consistent with her desire to live freely and fully, by her own standards. Not only has she lived beyond her prognosis, but she is cancer-free.

I recently saw Teresa P. at her annual checkup. At thirty-eight, she had been diagnosed with a lobular cancer with twenty-two positive lymph nodes. That was seventeen years ago. From the time of her diagnosis, she planned to survive the cancer in spite of the poor prognosis she was given.

Catherine K. had cancer recur in her lung four years after her initial diagnosis. That was fourteen years ago. After her relapse at age forty-two, she got her two boys off to college and developed a tremendously successful business. Melissa J. has survived her cancer for fourteen years. She has had a number of relapses that have not slowed her down. Two years ago she developed a lesion in her brain. She didn't miss a beat. Contrary to the traditional recommendation, she insisted that it be removed surgically, and she refused radiation. She decided to leave a fulfilling but stressful managerial position and take a job at her church teaching a senior citizens' Bible study group and helping with recreational event planning. She considered the job change not as acquiescing to her disease, but rather as a new phase in her life that allowed her to follow her heart.

Teri A.'s situation at diagnosis was serious. She was fifty and came to the emergency room with progressive shortness of breath. She was found to have nodules throughout both her lungs. The doctors were hopeful that the cause was an infection, but the diagnosis turned out to be breast cancer that had spread from a deep lesion in her left breast. She was transferred to the ICU and started chemotherapy. She immediately improved. Her only wish at that time was to see her first grandchild born. That was thirteen years ago. She has continued in treatment, as appropriate. I recently saw Teri and she invited me to her grandson's junior high school graduation.

I am fortunate that my patients remind me every day that life itself is a miracle. Each of us has been given a supreme gift to use at our discretion. Honoring that gift sometimes seems to be impossible. Yet our patients teach us that it is not just the grand gesture or big decisions which honor this gift, but the quiet decisions of individuals struggling to live their lives as authentically as possible that make the miracle.

∂ 14 ∂

Life with Breast Cancer

My barn having burned to the ground, I can now see the
moon.

—Old Taoist saying

Some of the significant changes you will have as a cancer patient are,
of course, physical in nature. You may lose a breast, or part of one.
Chemotherapy may cause you to lose your hair or gain weight. These
changes in appearance may affect how you feel as a woman. The purpose of this chapter is to address these and other issues relating to your
quality of life—body image, sexuality, and femininity.

The extent of the differences you experience will depend on the
treatment you'll require, your life stage, and on how proactive you are
in addressing the changes. If you are, for example, in a stable, supportive relationship and are beyond childbearing, these changes may
not be as disruptive as they might be for the woman who is single, premenopausal, and requires chemotherapy or ovarian suppression. Your
life may be drastically affected for a period of time. Besides the physical scars and altered body image, many women will have alterations
in their sexuality. Treatment may lead to ovarian suppression and a
lowering of hormone levels. This may cause a lack of sexual desire as
well as changes in vaginal mucosa leading to dryness and discomfort

during intercourse. With chemotherapy many women will lose their hair temporarily and there may be some body weight gain. The side effects must be assessed against the increased chance of being cured with the treatment. *It is important to keep in mind that, except for the physical scars, most if not all of these changes are temporary.*

Concerns about sexuality may not seem so important when viewed alongside survival, but as you get further away from the immediate crisis of the diagnosis and initiation of treatment, these quality-of-life issues become much more important. As you may already be aware, many physicians will not address physical, sexual, and emotional issues secondary to breast cancer treatment. Focused upon saving the patient's life, most physicians do not consider the long-term side effects of treatment. Often the patient is followed, after her "cancer treatment" is over, by her primary care physician, who may not be familiar with these effects or consider them his or hers to manage. In addition, some women feel reluctant to mention these areas of distress for fear of being embarrassed or appearing ungrateful.

Scarring

Unfortunately, there is no way to avoid physical scars from breast cancer. Clearly the paramount issue with breast cancer surgery is to remove the cancer with clear margins (that is, the cancer is removed completely, with an uninvolved area of normal breast between the cancer and the edge of the specimen). Often this can be accomplished with minimal change in the appearance of the breast. The amount of breast alteration depends on the size and location of the cancer, but also can depend a great deal on the skill and technique of the breast surgeon. Surgeons can create scars that follow the skin contours and will over time leave minimal deformity. If significant tissue is removed, the surgeon can move adjacent breast tissue to fill in the cavity. If mastectomy is required, many surgeons will leave as much skin as

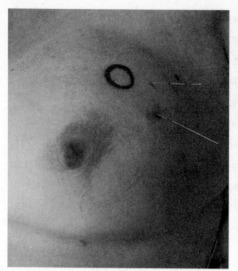 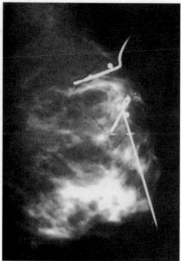

FIGURE 14.1   FIGURE 14.2

possible for optimal reconstruction. All too often, with the crisis of the diagnosis, surgery is performed without proper planning. This can lead to improperly placed incisions and often ends in the need for a second or third surgery. One of the major advantages of a preoperative needle biopsy diagnosis is that the proper surgery can usually be performed in one session. For most mammographically detected cancers, this requires the cooperation of the radiologist and pathologist. Ironically, most mammographically found cancers cannot be felt. The surgeon must therefore depend on the radiologist to identify the portion of the breast involved with the cancer. This is done by bracketing that area with wires that are inserted into the breast tissue to indicate the location of the suspicious mass. Often more than one of these wires is placed (see figures 14.1 and 14.2). This gives a better chance of removing the cancer with a clear area around it. If only one wire is placed, the surgeon usually removes the cancer with the localizing wire, but often the cancer is too close to the edge of the removed tissue to be considered to have a safe (clear) margin. If the radiologist puts in two or three wires and brackets the cancer, the surgeon has an excellent chance of removing the cancer with adequate clear surrounding tissue. When this is accomplished, follow-up radiation treatment may not be required. This depends on the individual woman's situation.

Once the specimen is out, it can be X-rayed to make sure the cancer is in the specimen. Several times a year I will see a woman (usually in second opinion) who had a biopsy she was told was benign but which was in fact cancerous. This becomes apparent when we review the mammograms and then the biopsy specimen and discover that the highly suspicious area seen on the films does not match up with the biopsy specimen seen under the microscope. Usually what has happened is that the wrong area of breast was removed and an X ray was not taken of the specimen to confirm that the abnormal area was removed. When we repeat the mammogram, the abnormality is still present on the film. I occasionally see a case where a surgeon thinks he or she doesn't need the help of the radiologist to localize the tumor and can find the tumor without guidance. This results in a greater loss of breast tissue and often incomplete removal, or "dirty margins." The bottom line is that if you have a choice, make sure the surgeon is planning to collaborate and is using his or her colleagues in radiology and pathology to give you not only the most complete breast cancer surgery available but the least deforming to you. Even utilizing the state of the art in technology and the expertise of the physicians involved, there can be a need for re-excision. Your surgeon will do his or her best to balance concern for conserving as much breast tissue as possible and achieving complete removal of the tumor. In addition, while much can be visualized through breast imaging, it may not comprehensively reveal all areas of tumor involvement. This can be known only after excision, when the specimen is reviewed by the pathologist.

The decision about where and how to operate will depend on the location of the cancer in your breast. Approximately two-thirds of cancers are in the upper outer quadrant of the breast. Incisions in this quadrant give the best cosmetic result because there is more tissue with which to work. Removal of even a large amount of tissue from this location usually does not disrupt the symmetry of the breast. If the cancer is in the center of the breast, a peri-areolar (around the areola or nipple) scar is cosmetically optimal. Cancers below the nipple, in the lower quadrants, can change the symmetry and leave the nipple-areolar complex not at the same level as that of the opposite breast. This can be further worsened by radiation. Cancers located directly behind the nipple sometimes require the nipple areolar complex to be removed with the cancer. In this case, I often feel it is better to do a skin-sparing mastectomy, particularly if radiation is necessary. The skin-sparing mastectomy will allow avoidance of radiation and usually gives a better cosmetic result with reconstruction.

If the cancer is in the upper inner quadrant, there may be increased risk of scarring and deformity. This quadrant has the least volume of breast tissue and is most visible in low-cut clothing. If the cancer is somewhat central, sometimes incision can be made around the areola and a tunnel can be created to remove the cancer with clear margins. The scar is semicircular at the border of the areola, and often after a year or so the scar is completely invisible. Plastic surgeons also use this technique to put in augmentation implants.

If you are newly diagnosed, you may think that the whole subject is not important when you are dealing with a possibly life-threatening illness. It is appropriate for you to be concerned about survival first but also about achieving good long-term cosmetic results and to actively seek both of these goals.

As I discussed previously, it is sometimes advantageous to give systemic therapy prior to surgery. Though the reasons for treating in this manner are not primarily cosmetic, the procedure usually has a much better cosmetic result than if the surgery is done first, followed by systemic therapy in the traditional way—because less tissue needs to be removed to give clear margins after the chemotherapy shrinks the cancer.

Mastectomy

The loss of a breast or breasts affects women in different ways. Many factors can complicate a woman's process of coping with this loss. Age at the time of diagnosis is one. A woman in the second half of her life often has different issues around the loss of a breast than a woman who is in her late twenties or thirties. Life situation and the presence of a partner is also an issue. Women who are not in a relationship and desire to be often have major concerns about their attractiveness and desirability to a future partner. The breast is an organ that has received a fair amount of "psychic attention" in our culture. It is an organ of nurturance in childhood and a focus of sensuality and sexuality from adolescence onward. Women, unfortunately, all too often describe their breasts as a primary factor in their assessment of their sexual desirability.

Women who seem to have the most difficult time with mastectomy are those who are heavily invested in their physical appearance and its contribution to their self-worth and self-esteem. Women who have had implant enhancement surgery prior to their breast cancer experience often fall into this category. These women are aware that plastic surgery can positively change their appearance. This knowledge is helpful, however, when considering mastectomy. Whether to remove a breast is a very difficult decision to make, particularly in this day and age when women are often given choices regarding surgical intervention. I find it useful to arrange a meeting between the patient and a woman who has been through the process and has returned to a satisfying life after breast cancer. This is particularly helpful for very young women, who are often devastated at diagnosis and feel their life is over, even when they understand they will survive the disease.

Hormonal Changes

One of the unanticipated changes that many women will experience as a side effect of treatment is hormonal change. For the postmenopausal woman who is on replacement estrogen, her physicians will often recommend that she discontinue her hormone replacement therapy (HRT) if her breast cancer is estrogen receptor–positive. This can acutely add to her distress at a time when she is required to address the cancer crisis and the necessary treatment decisions. When a woman who has been on HRT for some time suddenly discontinues her estrogen, she will have a rapid falling off of her hormone levels and will experience symptoms of menopause. These may include hot flashes, a decrease in sexual desire, mood swings, and sleep disturbance. We think that some of these symptoms are a result of serotonin depletion. Over time, the lack of estrogen will affect the vaginal lining, causing thinning and a decrease in lubrication. This can lead to difficulty with sexual function, mainly discomfort during intercourse as well as an increased likelihood of urinary tract infection. Premenopausal women may experience many of these same symptoms when their ovarian function is suppressed as a side effect of chemotherapy or medications that directly stop estrogen production.

Many women are willing to undergo these changes and make adjustments in the quality of their life if the result is an increased likelihood of curing their cancer. Women are often not forewarned by their physicians as to what to expect. Much can be done to relieve symptoms and to make the process more tolerable. Unfortunately, many physicians do not address these issues until the symptoms are so severe that they are causing major distress.

I do not believe it is necessary to take the postmenopausal woman off her HRT abruptly. I feel it is safe and makes more sense to taper the HRT over a four- to six-week period. This will avert major or severe mood disturbances associated with acute withdrawal at the critical time of coping with the crisis of breast cancer. The use of the herbal remedy St. John's wort, the amino acid precursor 5-hydroxytryptophan, or low-dose antidepressants is particularly helpful. The SSRI class of antidepressants, such as Prozac, Zoloft, and Paxil, at half the usual dosage given for depressions can help alleviate hot flashes and mood disturbance.

Vaginal dryness can be diminished by applying long-acting water-soluble lubricants such as Replens or Astroglide. The use of vaginal estrogen cream can also lead to a significant amount of estrogen absorption into the system. We now know that the skin and mucosa have the ability to rapidly absorb medication. This was recently dramatically demonstrated when a man came to one of our breast centers with a complaint of rapid enlargement of his breasts, a condition we call gynecomastia. It turned out that his wife was taking estrogen cream for vaginal mucosa thinning and dryness. She misunderstood the directions and was using the cream as a lubricant for sex. Her husband was absorbing a large amount of estrogen during intercourse, and it was causing his breast tissue to swell.

Fortunately, we now have a safe solution for the vaginal atrophy associated with estrogen deprivation. It involves the use of a small silastic ring (similar in texture to a diaphragm) impregnated with estrogen, which is very slowly released. Tissue levels of estrogen have been measured before and during the use of this ring, and the amount of estrogen that is absorbed is very small. The ring remains in the vagina for three months and fits high in the vaginal vault around the cervix. For women who have had a hysterectomy, it may be a problem to get the device to stay in place. A set of exercises called Kegels may help to keep this device well situated within the vagina and aid in the prevention of urinary incontinence. The majority of women using this device have experienced marked relief from their symptoms of estrogen deprivation. (See also chapter 15.)

Sex and Chemotherapy

For a majority of newly diagnosed women, sexual intimacy is put on the back burner during this period of crisis. With surgery and wound dressings and post-op discomfort, sex is usually not an immediate concern. However, it certainly becomes a concern, and the real problem often begins after the physical wounds have healed. There is a measurable decrease in sex drive due to the hormonal changes associated with chemotherapy or the antiestrogen drug tamoxifen. Another part of the chemotherapy effect is the general malaise associated with the known toxicity of the drugs. There is usually complete hair loss on the head and body, and the mucous membranes in the mouth and vagina are sensitive and tender. Sexual desire or libido is clearly diminished if not absent altogether. It is important to note that libido and sexuality are complex and are not completely dependent on estrogen. Clearly, postmenopausal women who are not on HRT can have normal libidos. In fact, libido seems better correlated to testosterone than estrogen levels. Testosterone is produced by the adrenal glands and the ovaries. Young women who have had their ovaries removed often suffer a loss of libido. This can be corrected by giving small amounts of testosterone, in cream form, small oral doses, or a timed-release testosterone pellet inserted just below the skin surface.

The mechanism by which libido is impaired with tamoxifen use is not clear. Patients given tamoxifen often have testosterone levels that are slightly low to normal. Again, a small amount of testosterone sometimes helps, and the general consensus is that it is safe as far as the breast cancer recurrence risk is concerned. Certainly a large component of sexuality is feeling good about yourself and not being depressed. In this regard, many of the suggestions that are made in chapter 12 apply. Exercise and diet are extremely important, and the use of medication can help. It also helps to have a loving and understanding partner.

Chemotherapy and tamoxifen to prevent metastatic disease is given for a finite period of time. Chemotherapy lasts on average three to six months with another three to six months for the body to recover. Some premenopausal women will go into permanent menopause from chemotherapy. The chance of this depends on age and the intensity or aggressiveness of the chemotherapy. The closer the patient is to natural menopause, the more likely chemotherapy will put her into it. If premature menopause is caused by chemotherapy, should a woman be put on hormone replacement? This is a complex issue, and I think it depends on the breast cancer and whether it is promoted by hormones or not. We will consider putting a postmenopausal woman on HRT after chemotherapy if her tumor is not hormone-sensitive and if her quality of life is significantly negatively affected. If the tumor is hormone-sensitive, tamoxifen for three to five years is generally recommended, and HRT should be avoided.

The recommended length of tamoxifen treatment is a matter of controversy. Five years is the standard and two years seems to be insufficient. The optimal period is between three and five years. There is evidence that new compounds called aromatase inhibitors may be more effective than tamoxifen in postmenopausal women and have fewer side effects. Aromatase inhibitors are ineffective, however, when the ovaries are producing estrogen or a woman is receiving replacement hormones. Women receiving aromatase inhibitors also have many of the side effects of estrogen deprivation. At some point, adjuvant therapy will be discontinued—chemotherapy at six months and tamoxifen or an aromatase inhibitor at three to five years. Most women who have a significant survival benefit from chemotherapy will accept the estrogen deprivation associated with these treatments, albeit with trepidation. The good news about tamoxifen is that it can be discontinued at any time and within three weeks its effects are gone. Many of the hormonal side effects of tamoxifen are helped by the approaches discussed in chapter 12. We occasionally recommend low-dose progesterone and testosterone to treat hot flashes and decreased libido when these side effects are exceptionally debilitating. Exercise and yoga are helpful for many women. Herbs and soy can help with hot flashes, although some laboratory data indicate that specific plant or phyto estrogens—soy, for example—can (rarely) stimulate some breast cancers. For this reason these should be used with caution.

Fertility and Reproduction

One of the most significant quality-of-life issues premenopausal patients grapple with is fertility and reproduction. Approximately 25 percent of women who develop breast cancer do so in their reproductive years. Breast cancer in this age group tends to be somewhat more aggressive and often requires systemic therapy of some type. By the time this therapy has been completed, a certain percentage of these women will be beyond reproductive ability due to age. Added to this group are the women who have premature menopause from the therapy itself. Most younger women who receive chemotherapy will have some disruption of their hormone cycling. This is manifested by symptoms of menopause such as hot flashes or vaginal dryness. The menstrual cycling may change, and many women may temporarily cease having their period. This is usually a six- to twelve-month process, and normalcy will likely resume by twelve months. The chance of a woman in her thirties losing her reproductive capacity due to chemotherapy and the possible addition of tamoxifen is less than 30 percent. For women in their forties the chance of chemically induced ovarian failure rises. The drugs must somehow affect remaining eggs and follicle development to some degree. A woman is born with a fixed number of eggs in her two ovaries. When she reaches puberty and begins to menstruate, eggs begin to form follicles on a thirty-day or so cycle. With each cycle, a few eggs are stimulated by pituitary hormones and begin to work their way to the surface of the ovaries. The surrounding supporting cells, what we call stromal cells, make hormones that prepare the uterus for the fertilized egg that will be extruded from the surface of an ovary and picked up by a fallopian tube and carried to the uterus for implantation.

For the woman who wants to have a baby after breast cancer, the reality that this might not be possible because of the side effects of chemotherapy sets up its own grieving process. A pressing question is whether it is ever safe to have a baby after breast cancer. The answer to this is at once simple and complex. The simple answer is, it is safe if the woman is cured. The complex part is that we don't know for sure who is cured. We know that a pregnancy does not cause recurrence. The risk is that if a woman is not cured, a pregnancy could theoretically accelerate a relapse via the hormone stimulation of pregnancy. In my experience this is a rare occurrence; I have seen it happen on only two occasions in twenty-five years of caring for women with breast cancer. I have personally taken care of dozens of women who have had children after a breast cancer diagnosis and treatment.

Many women ask me if there is anything that can be done to protect ovarian function from cytotoxic chemotherapy. Most oncologists are not employing strategies that might protect the ovaries. In fact, I don't think it is even considered by many oncologists. It is again a situation where one specialist, in this case an oncologist, is not collaborating with the gynecologist who specializes in endocrine function and fertility. I have heard oncologists say at meetings that one of the benefits of chemotherapy is ovarian suppression, which may have a beneficial effect on survival in estrogen-positive breast cancer. Although there is truth to this belief and data to support it, there are better ways to achieve ovarian suppression than poisoning the ovaries with non-discriminatory chemotherapies. As I have stated before, chemotherapy is overutilized in low-grade hormone-positive breast cancer. The mainstay of systemic treatment for this less aggressive breast cancer is hormonal manipulation through estrogen-depriving drugs. One of the ways to protect the ovaries is not to use chemotherapy if it is not indicated. If chemotherapy is necessary, there are several ways to shield or protect the ovaries from the damaging effect of the drugs. The simplest approach is to put the ovaries at rest by suppressing ovulation. This can easily be done using either the LHRH agonist or the LHRH antagonist drugs. These drugs interfere with the pituitary's ability to make FSH (follicle-stimulating hormones), which leads to ovulation and estrogen production.

I am not aware of any controlled studies comparing women in which there has been an attempt to protect the ovarian function in this way to women treated in the conventional manner. Another approach would be to remove the ovary or part of an ovary, freeze it, and then replace it after therapy is over. There is some literature on the subject, but I am not aware of any institution that is attempting to do this in any organized trial or fashion. Nor am I aware as of this writing of a baby being born from a transplanted ovary.

If the primary consideration is to preserve eggs for procreation, an obvious approach is to harvest and store eggs. There has been tremendous progress in this area of medicine using microsurgery and ovarian stimulation with hormones. Unfortunately, the viability rate for harvested eggs and their ability to be fertilized later is not high, so it is not a sure way of success. The research reflects a 10 percent success rate with unfertilized eggs. A more successful approach is storing fertilized eggs for later implantation into either the donor or a surrogate. This method requires hormone stimulation for ovulation and harvest. It delays chemotherapy for a number of weeks but could be taking place prior to chemotherapy during the breast surgery phase of treatment. This can be especially risky in women whose tumors are estrogen receptor–positive and should be undertaken with extreme caution.

New technology in reproductive endocrinology and genetic cloning will have a major impact on the ability of young women with cured breast cancer to have children. It will require oncologists to work with other specialists. Physicians also have to realize that breast cancer is a heterogeneous disease and that women with the type of breast cancer that is not related to hormones can be treated differently from women with other subtypes.

Today, 80 percent of women with breast cancer are cured. Once we have done what we can, we need to support women as they pursue their lives and as they continue to recover. There is much we can do to promote physical recovery. We need to encourage them to live with gusto and to support them in doing so.

Life after breast cancer is life with a body that is new to you—forever changed by treatment. You will have different life choices ahead because of your breast cancer, new avenues to explore and decisions to make. You will move forward and reclaim your life.

❧ 15 ❧

Renewing Your Sexuality

Up the Down Slope

Come to the edge.
No, we will fall.

Come to the edge.
No, we will fall.

They came to the edge.
He pushed them, and they flew.

—Guillaume Apollinaire

A woman with newly diagnosed breast cancer approaches her sexuality changed by her breast cancer experience. These changes affect both your relationship to yourself and your relationship with your partner. Because each newly diagnosed woman's situation is different, and your relationship is unique, some of the issues I will raise in this chapter may not apply to you and your loved one. I hope some of the suggestions will prove valuable as you strive to achieve a new awareness of your own sexual needs and feelings and to communicate this positively to your partner.

Although the breast cancer has occurred in your body, it has also affected your partner. You will be dealing with changes in your body as well as in your feelings and body image. In order for your partner to understand these changes, you will need to be able to describe them and, more important, discuss how they'll affect the physical and sexual life that you share. Ideally, you will learn new coping skills both as an individual and as a couple.

The most obvious impact of treatment for breast cancer on sexuality is in the area of body image. One of the very first treatment decisions you will be asked to make will involve the issue of local control of the cancer. There are usually two options, breast conservation or mastectomy. In some cases, there is really little choice. In these cases mastectomy is the safer and sometimes the only option to optimize cure. A second opinion is always helpful to settle any questions about the risk or benefit of a recommendation for mastectomy. It is important to keep in mind that, with a mastectomy, there is always the option of breast reconstruction. Insurance will almost always pay for this. Reconstruction can be done at the time of the original operation or later, depending on the circumstances. It may facilitate your decision making to coordinate your surgical and reconstructive surgery consultations prior to any actual surgical intervention. In this way you will be fully informed about reconstruction options and your general surgeon and reconstructive surgeon can confer and agree on their surgical approach.

Regardless of whether a mastectomy or lumpectomy is done, there is always a sense of loss and grief. The extent of this grief depends on many circumstances, including the intervention decided upon, your age, and how significant your breasts have been to your self-esteem and sexuality. If you're single, then you'll have to establish a new relationship with your changed body by yourself and decide how and when you share that with a partner. If you are in a long-term relationship, your basic communication with your partner concerning your body and sexuality is, ideally, already established. However, even the best and clearest communication styles can be enriched. The breast cancer experience is an opportunity to deepen the intimacy of your communication with and connection to your partner as well as to increase your level of sexual satisfaction.

Following the surgery, you may feel anxiety or fear about your appearance and your scars. You will want to assess for yourself how involved you want or need your partner to be in your after-care. In general, the sooner you begin to acknowledge and accept the changes in your body, the sooner you will pursue and establish a new sense of normalcy about your body and sexual contact. Your doctor, it is hoped, will encourage this. Yet, some women are hesitant to involve their partner at this point. This is a process of self-acceptance, adjustment, and then, as you feel more familiar with the changes, sharing with your partner. For some women, their partner's acceptance of their altered physical appearance is a critical precursor to their self-acceptance. Other women must come to terms with their changes alone before they can share them with a partner. Do what is right for you. You know your partner and your relationship, and you will make the best decision as to when and how much to include your partner in your recovery.

Your physical healing will not occur overnight. You will want to be careful to note the manner in which healing and change continue to occur, particularly in the first year after surgery. Scarring generally diminishes as your body continues to heal, and you'll want to expect this as well as appreciate the process. Although your body will never be the same, your intimacy—emotional, physical, and mental—has the potential to be even greater as you share the losses with your partner and explore new areas of pleasure. If your breasts were a signficant focus of arousal and pleasure for you and/or your partner, their loss will need to be addressed and additional erogenous areas explored.

Obviously, physical touch is important, especially if your relationship has been very physically affectionate and/or sexual in the past. It is a time when you may feel unattractive; physical touch and what we refer to as "nondemand" pleasure (meaning pleasurable touch without any demand) may be reassuring. Again, communication is the key.

Asking specifically for the contact you want and tactfully setting clear boundaries around what does not feel comfortable will help you and your partner to approach the changes in your body and sexuality with greater confidence.

In addition to surgery, you may be undergoing other treatments that will impact your general sense of well-being as well as your sexuality. If you receive chemotherapy, it may reduce your energy and vigor and cause hair loss. You may feel more fatigued than you have ever felt in your life, but it will not be the fatigue you feel at the end of a day's work or after a workout at the gym. Where previously you may have rebounded quickly from such stressors, you will not be able to do so after chemotherapy. This may be frustrating to you and to your partner. Remember, this is new territory for both of you. Studies show that what is called "cancer-related fatigue" is not the same as the garden variety fatigue which most well people experience. You *will* recover, and your ability to alternate physical stress, as you tolerate it, with periods of rest is critically important to your recovery.

As part of your treatment protocol, hormone replacement therapy may be stopped. Chemotherapy may also cause the ovaries to slow down estrogen production temporarily or permanently, leading to menopausal symptoms. Whether it be the result of stopping hormone replacement therapy or of undergoing chemotherapy, a lack of estrogen leads to thinning of mucous membranes, particularly in the vagina, as well as a diminishment or loss of sexual interest or desire.

If you have desire for sexual contact, you may still experience some discomfort with intercourse because of these changes in the vagina and surrounding tissue. It is important to use vaginal lubricants and, when you are ready, proceed gradually with an understanding of these changes. However, sex is rarely a high priority for women in treatment. Exploring your renewed sexuality needs to be a gradual process— beginning and ending where you feel comfortable and increasing over time.

A number of studies that have looked at quality of life after breast cancer treatment show that sexual discomfort appears to be more prevalent in women who have undergone chemotherapy. Dr. Patricia Ganz at UCLA surveyed almost a thousand women who were, on average, six years post-treatment. She compared their quality of life before and after treatment. A vast majority of women had equal or better quality of life in virtually all areas measured, save one—sexual function. Women who had chemotherapy continued to have problems with lubrication and pain even years after treatment. I suspect part of the pain of sexual contact is due to vaginal atrophy from lack of estrogen. Using vaginal lubricants and/or a silastic vaginal ring that fits up around the cervix and emits small amounts of estrogen can make a huge difference in allowing a woman to have positive sexual experiences during and after treatment. The silastic ring takes several weeks before its effects are noticed. It is changed every three months, and usually neither the woman nor her partner is aware that it is in place. In addition, some women find that Kegel exercises, which are commonly prescribed by gynecologists for urinary incontinence, help in keeping pelvic floor muscles firm and intact, thus facilitating sexual arousal and satisfaction.

For many women the process of breast cancer diagnosis and treatment impairs their ability and willingness to invest in the body as a source of pleasure and trust. They have been through so much that is unpleasant and/or painful that they have lost the memory of a body that reliably and predictably brings them pleasurable experiences of any kind, let alone sexual pleasure. If this is true for you, then you will want to systematically focus your awareness on the experiences that remain pleasurable for you even as you introduce yourself to new experiences. You will need to anchor your body in both the memory and the anticipation of physical pleasure and to separate out the unpleasant experiences that are part of the treatment process. You will want to cultivate an active pursuit of pleasure.

I have, briefly, described many physical and sexual changes that occur as a result of a breast cancer diagnosis. There has been a lot of progress in understanding and managing the sexual consequences of breast cancer treatment. Although the issues may sound daunting, *do not give up*. If you encounter difficulty, talk with your oncologist, gynecologist, and/or psychotherapist about your concerns. They *can* be worked through, if you are willing to take on the challenge. You will go through many losses, but a quality sexual life need not be one of them. Through treatment and beyond, breast cancer survivors have an opportunity to reinvest in their sexual lives in a conscious manner, pursuing with renewed vigor and appreciation an expression of their sexual identity that best meets their needs as well as the needs of their partner. *Take it on*.

∞ 16 ∞

Ikiru: To Live

A bird doesn't sing because it has an answer, it sings because
it has a song to sing.

—Maya Angelou

Few events rival the existential crisis of a life-threatening illness.
Even with the smallest mammographically detected breast cancer,
nothing is ever the same. You are forced to look at your mortality,
even if for just an instant. In that glimpse, however brief, is the opportunity to review your life and how you are living it. The specter of
death sits perched on your shoulder, a reminder that time is limited
and that you, and no one else, are in charge of your remaining hours,
days, and years. Though we cannot undo past decisions that have
proven painful, we can learn from those decisions and commit to honoring that learning in changed behavior in the future. Each and every
moment we have the opportunity to let go of the past and to begin
again. Your breast cancer diagnosis is not the end of the road but a
profound reminder that each day you have the chance to write anew
on the slate of your life—to *live*.

As a medical student, I experienced this existential frontier as an
observer. While completing my internship I had the opportunity to

see a Japanese film entitled *Ikiru*. Made in 1952, it was directed by the famous Japanese filmmaker Akira Kurosawa. *Ikiru* is about an ordinary man, an aging bureaucrat named Kanji Watanabe, who develops terminal stomach cancer (not an uncommon cancer in Japan). His life is joyless, a string of days and years of existence without meaning or passion. There is a hint that much earlier in his life he had a commitment to values and ideals, but that this commitment had long been lost. The banality of his existence, together with the knowledge of his terminal illness, ignites in him a quest to engage in something—anything—that will be meaningful to him and satisfy his soul's need to create. As he seeks such an object or project, he stumbles, falls, and rights himself. The pressure of knowing he has limited time urges him on. He makes a miraculous transformation. After almost forty years of pushing papers, he takes on the project of creating a park in the middle of a crowded Japanese city. With this new passion, his life becomes meaningful to him again. In his last six months of life, he experiences more joy and fulfillment than in his entire previous sixty years.

There is an unforgettable scene in which Watanabe is on a swing in his newly created park. It is snowing and he is singing, "Life is short. . . ." His face reflects absolute joy and peace as the snow falls gently around him and he swings like a child. His project is complete and he has a clear sense of fulfillment and wholeness that is riveting. I have not seen the film in thirty years, but it had a profound effect on my career and my life. It reminded me that the quality of living is what is important. For those of us in the healing profession, it is certainly enough to ease pain, relieve symptoms, and sometimes "cure" a "disease." It is a breathtaking bonus when we have the opportunity to witness a transformation in which the crisis has led to an awakening, an integration of the mind, body, and spirit that brings true peace.

In *Ikiru*, Watanabe lived fifty-nine years, or more than three hundred thousand waking hours, of a banal, miserable existence. His life, 99 percent over, down to the final two thousand hours, was suddenly transformed into one of meaning and fulfillment—by his definition. Life itself provides daily reminders of the opportunities to live it meaningfully. We hope that we heed the call because what we observe about the end of life is that answering this call to meaning seems to be all that really matters.

A second lesson I learned from *Ikiru* is that even the seemingly impossible can happen, and that illness can be the agent of change. Watanabe could have chosen to close himself off from the possibilities for meaningful transformation, out of despair and a lifetime of numbed, unfulfilled longing. He doesn't. Instead he does something wondrous. When many would find it prudent to simply shut down their lives, he opened his to the inspiration of *what might be* today— while he still exists—and this choice changed everything.

You must decide for yourself how you will find or affirm that which is meaningful to you in your life. We see breast cancer survivors who become lifelong peer mentors to newly diagnosed patients, some who love to travel and make it a top priority to take the trips they dream of, and some who decide to seek a new job or more education in order to fulfill their needs more deeply. For still others, it is a less obvious but equally powerful inner reorientation, realized as they remind themselves consciously that, in what counts most to them, they already have their heart's desires. This is your journey—you are already on a path. Is it the path that your soul calls you to travel?

As an oncologist I see the *Ikiru* phenomenon—or call to transformation—in real life. I see patients who have always lived their lives honoring the need for meaningful activity and others who despair that fulfillment may never be theirs.

Occasionally I will give a seminar to newly diagnosed patients and their loved ones. It is obviously a difficult and emotional time, to which you can probably personally relate. I ask them to play a game with me. I want them to imagine that they have three healthy years remaining in their life to do anything they want. There are 15,330 waking hours—or three years—to spend in any way they wish in the context of their present life. What I mean is that they can't imagine being someone else. There is no way to escape; the end is inevitable. I ask them to write out their remaining life plan. Three years is longer than the time given to the bureaucrat in *Ikiru*. It is long enough to plant a garden and see it bloom two, maybe three times. It's long enough to write a book or a volume of poetry or to reconcile with a lost brother. It's long enough to make a difference in the life of a child. It's long enough to learn a new language or experience another culture or understand one's own culture better.

The exercise involves taking control and living every hour by choice and not by default. Life is a string of minutes and hours. It is the summation of small interactions and events of which each of us is the director. It is living one's life making active choices, not reacting to the world around you. How many of us spend our lives doing things we would rather not be doing, with people we would rather not be with, or whom we haven't taken the time to really know?

Psychologists and philosophers agree that one of the most anxiety-provoking things about life is that we don't know when we will die. Human beings want to be in control, and yet this is the one area over which we have no control. To actually acknowledge that you, like everyone, have a finite period to live, brings to the fore the question: Do you want to live differently? Clearly if you are living in an abusive relationship, or working at a job that is unrewarding, you might make an immediate decision for change. The majority of women faced with breast cancer make subtler changes that can lead to a profound transformation.

The knowledge that your remaining time is limited can lead to myriad decisions that can greatly enrich your life. These decisions may seem small, like spending a few extra minutes watching children play in the park, or getting up early and watching the sunrise, or giving your child or grandchild a positive affirmation. There is a reorientation to what is in charge of your life—your time. This should be the gift of breast cancer: a wake-up call to live your remaining life with gusto, doing what you want to do minute to minute, working actively to find beauty, meaning, purpose, an affirmation of values in that which you previously found meaningless—or releasing yourself from it. The gift is a release to live—*Ikiru*. The lesson of *Ikiru* is that anyone can make the transformation. *Hear the call.*

A Final Thought

Life is a promise; fulfill it.
—Mother Teresa

If there is one abiding concept that unifies this book, it is the notion that breast cancer requires that you be treated as a whole person— body, mind, emotions, and spirit. Optimal treatment is the treatment that is best for you, not just the unique manifestation of cancer that has arisen in your body, but also the inherent emotional, spiritual, and mental reorientation the crisis ignites. Change in you and your experience of what is important to you *will occur*. The question is whether or not you will determine the direction of that change or simply be the passive receiver of it.

You need to remember that you are not alone. There are hundreds of thousands of women who have preceded you. And each one of them has had to integrate her experience of diagnosis and treatment into the larger context of her life. These women have a story to tell, just as you do. And with each telling, you will come to understand more deeply the true nature of the changes that have occurred in you. You will, most likely, be cured—yes, *cured*—but it takes time for this reality to impact a mind, heart, body, and soul that have known terror.

But the answer to terror is not blind hope; it is an understanding and appreciation of the mystery of life. It is this mystery that tells us that as much as medicine can define an illness and treat it, medicine cannot tell us who will be cured and who will recur. It cannot tell us who will have a fire ignited in her soul as a result of her experience and who will not. In this space, created by the crisis, we are given the opportunity to experience what it means to be naked to our core; to reclaim our birthright in a renewed sense of unadulterated joy and awareness of spirit. Some will discover it as a call to prayer; for others it will be the breathtaking sight of their sleeping child; for yet others, the greeting of a new sunrise. It is a state of grace for which there can be no road map; the journey is as unique as each individual.

In her book *A Short Guide to a Happy Life*, Anna Quindlen describes her journey of transformation after her mother's death:

> I learned to love the journey, not the destination. I learned that this is not a dress rehearsal, and that today is the only guarantee you get.
>
> I learned to look at all the good in the world and to try to give some back, because I believed in it completely and utterly. And I tried to do that, in part, by telling others what I had learned. . . . By telling them this: Consider the lilies of the field. Look at the fuzz on a baby's ear. Read in the back-yard with the sun on your face. Learn to be happy. And think of life as a terminal illness, because, if you do, you will live it with joy and passion as it ought to be lived.

Breast cancer reminds us that life is terminal. *Live well.*

References

Chapter 1: You Are in Charge

Link, J. S., *The Breast Cancer Survival Manual*. New York: Henry Holt/Owl Books, 1998.

Chapter 2: Demystifying the Disease

Tabar, L., C. J. G. Fagerberg, A. Gad, et al., Reduction in Mortality from Breast Cancer after Mass Screening with Mammography. *Lancet* 1 (1985): 829–832.

Chapter 3: Look before You Leap

Abeloff, M. D., Oncology and Hematology: An Internet Resource Guide. www.eMedguides.com, Inc. May 2001–April 2002.

Giuliano, A. E., D. M. Kirgan, J. M. Guenther, et al., Lymphatic Mapping and Sentinel Lymphadenectomy for Breast Cancer. *Annals of Surgery* 220 (1994): 391–401.

Schirrmeister, H., T. Kuhn, A. Guhlmann, et al., Fluorine—18 2-Deoxy-2-Fluoro-D-Glucose PET in the Preoperative Staging of Breast Cancer: Comparison with Standard Staging Procedures. *European Journal of Nuclear Medicine* 28 (2001): 351–358.

Weinstein, S. P., S. G. Orel, R. Heller, et al., MR Imaging (MRI) of the Breast in Patients with Invasive Lobular Carcinoma. *American Journal of Roentgenology* 176 (2001): 399–406.

Yap, C. S., M. A. Seltzer, C. Schiepers, et al., Impact of Whole-Body 18F-FDG PET on Staging and Managing Patients with Breast Cancer: The Referring Physician's Perspective. *Journal of Nuclear Medicine* 42 (9) (September 2000): 1334–1337.

Chapter 4: Treating the Whole Woman

Weiss, B., *Message from the Masters: Tapping into the Power of Love*. New York, Warner Books, 2000, p. 178.

Chapter 5: Your Doctor Is Human, Too

Aring, C. D., Sympathy and Empathy. *Journal of the American Medical Association* 167 (4) (May 24, 1959): 448–452.
Stephens, L., Commencement Address delivered to the University of Southern California School of Medicine, Class of 1973. June 1973, Los Angeles, Calif.

Chapter 7: Saving Your Breast

Kushner, R., *Alternatives: New Developments in the War on Breast Cancer*. Cambridge, Mass., Kensington Press, 1984.

Chapter 8: Weighing the Risk

Brambilla, C., A. Escobedo, et al., Medical Castration with Zoladex: A Conservative Approach to Premenopausal Breast Cancer. *Tumori* 77 (2) (April 30, 1991): 145–150.
Mamounas, E. P., and B. Fisher, Preoperative (Neoadjuvant) Chemotherapy in Patients with Breast Cancer. *Seminars in Oncology* 28 (4) (August 2001): 389–399.
Matsumoto, M., M. Miyauchi, et al., Investigation of Menstruation Recovery after LH-RH Agonist Therapy for Premenopausal Patients with Breast Cancer. *Breast Cancer* 7 (3) (2000): 237–240.
Page, D. L., and B. A. Carter, Sentinel Lymph Nodes, Breast Cancer, and Pseudometastases. *Breast Diseases: A Year Book Quarterly* 12 (4) (2002): 362–363.

Chapter 9: The New Era: Genetics and Breast Cancer

Livingston, D. M., and R. Shivadasani, Toward Mechanism-Based Cancer Care. *Journal of the American Medical Association* 285 (5) (February 7, 2001): 588–593.

Macoska, J. A., The Progressing Clinical Utility of DNA Microarrays. *Cancer* 52 (1) (January/February 2002).

Rieger, P. T., *Biotherapy: A Comprehensive Overview*, 2nd ed. Sudbury, Mass.: Jones and Bartlett, 2001.

Chapter 10: The New Agents

Bazell, R., *Her-2: The Making of Herceptin, a Revolutionary Treatment for Breast Cancer.* New York: Random House, 1998.

Slamon, D. J., et al., Use of Chemotherapy plus a Monoclonal Antibody against Her-2 for Metastatic Breast Cancer That Overexpresses Her-2. *New England Journal of Medicine* 344 (11) (March 15, 2002): 783–792.

Chapter 12: The Mind Is a Powerful Thing

Preston, J. D., J. H. O'Neal, and M. C. Talaga, *Handbook of Clinical Psychopharmacology for Therapists.* Oakland, Calif.: New Harbinger Publications, 2000.

Richardson, E., Pharmacology of Antidepressants—Characteristics of the Ideal Drug. *Mayo Clinic Proceedings* 69 (1994):1069–1081.

Seiden, O., M.D., *5-HTP: The Serotonin Connection.* Roseville, Calif.: Prima Health, 1998.

Siegel, B. S., Love Medicine & Miracles. New York: Harper, 1990.

Skidmore-Roth, L., *Handbook of Herbs & Natural Supplements.* St. Louis, Mo.: Mosby-Year Book, 2001.

Spiegel, D., et al., Effect of Psychosocial Treatment on Survival of Patients with Metastatic Breast Cancer. *Lancet* 2 (8668) (1989): 888–891.

Weil, A., M.D., *Spontaneous Healing.* New York: Fawcett Columbine, 1995.

Yance, D. R., *Herbal Medicine, Healing and Cancer.* New Canaan, Conn.: Keats Publishing, 1999.

Chapter 13: Faith, Healing, and Miracles

Bruyere, R., *Wheels of Light: A Study of the Chakras*. New York: Simon & Schuster, 1989.

Davidson, S., Energy Magic—Visiting Rosalyn Bruyere. O, *The Oprah Magazine* (November 2001): 232–235.

Hirshberg, C., and M. Barasch, *Remarkable Recovery: What Extraordinary Healings Tell Us about Getting Well and Staying Well*. New York: Riverhead Books, 1995.

Hunt, V., *Infinite Mind: Science of Human Vibrations of Consciousness*. Malibu, Calif.: Malibu Publishing Company, 1989.

LeShan, L., *Cancer as a Turning Point*. New York: Plume, Penguin Books, 1989.

Moyers, B., *Healing and the Mind*. New York: Doubleday, 1993.

Simonton, O. C., and S. Mathews-Simonton, *Getting Well Again*. New York: Bantam Books, 1978.

Chapter 14: Life with Breast Cancer

Burstein, H. J., and E. P. Winer, Reproductive Issues in Breast Cancer Patients. *Diseases of the Breast Updates* 3 (1999).

Ginsburg, E. S., E. H. Yanushpolsky, and K. V. Jackson, In Vitro Fertilization for Cancer Patients and Survivors. *Fertility and Sterility* 75 (2001): 705–710.

Kutluk, O., and K. Economos, Endocrine Function and Oocyte Retrieval after Autologous Transplantation of Ovarian Cortical Strips to the Forearm. *Journal of the American Medical Association* 286 (12) (September 26, 2001).

Meirow, D., Reproduction Post-Chemotherapy in Young Cancer Patients. *Molecular and Cell Endocrinology* 169 (12) (November 27, 2000): 123–131.

O'Meara, E. S., M. A. Rossing, J. R. Daling, et al., Hormone Replacement Therapy after a Diagnosis of Breast Cancer in Relation to Recurrence and Mortality. *Journal of the National Cancer Institute* 93 (2001): 754–762.

Chapter 15: Renewing Your Sexuality

Ganz, P. A., K. A. Desmond, B. Leedham, J. H. Rowland, B. E. Meyerowitz, and T. R. Belin, Quality of Life in Long-Term Disease-Free Survivors of Breast Cancer: A Follow-up Study. *Journey of the National Cancer Institute* 94 (January 2, 2002).

Kahane, D. H., *No Less a Woman*. New York: Prentice-Hall, 1990.

Lange, V., *Be a Survivor*. Lange Productions, 1999.

Schover, L. R., Sexuality & Cancer: For the Woman Who Has Cancer and Her Partner. American Cancer Society, 1996 (call 800-ACS-2345).

Chapter 16: Ikiru: *To Live*

Dossey, L., *Meaning & Medicine*. New York: Bantam Books, 1991.

Murray, E., *"Ikiru": Ten Film Classics: A Re-Viewing*. New York: Frederick Ungar, 1978.

Spiegel, D., *Living beyond the Limits*. New York: Fawcett Columbine, Ballantine Books, 1994.

A Final Thought

Quindlen, A., *A Short Guide to a Happy Life*. New York: Random House, 2000.

Resources

NCI Designated Cancer Centers

ALABAMA
UAB *Comprehensive Cancer Center*
University of Alabama at
Birmingham
(Comprehensive Cancer Center)
1824 Sixth Avenue South, Room 237
Birmingham, AL 35293-3300
Tel: 205/934-5077
Fax: 205/975-7428
www.ccc.uab.edu

ARIZONA
Arizona Cancer Center
University of Arizona
(Comprehensive Cancer Center)
1501 North Campbell Avenue
Tucson, AZ 85724
Tel: 520/626-7925
Fax: 520/626-2284
www.azcc.arizona.edu

CALIFORNIA
The Burnham Institute
(Cancer Center)
10901 North Torrey Pines Road
LaJolla, CA 92037

Tel: 858/646-3132
Fax: 858/646-3184
www.burnham-inst.org

Cancer Center
Salk Institute
(Cancer Center)
10100 North Torrey Pines Road
LaJolla, CA 92037
Tel: 858/453-4100 X1386
Fax: 858/457-4765
www.salk.edu

Chao Family Comprehensive
Cancer Center
University of California at Irvine
(Comprehensive Cancer Center)
101 The City Drive
Room 406, Building 23, Route 81
Orange, CA 92868
Tel: 714/456-6310
Fax: 714/456-2240
www.ucihealth.com/cancer/

City of Hope National Medical Center
& Beckman Research Institute

(Comprehensive Cancer Center)
1500 East Duarte Road
Duarte, CA 91010-3000
Tel: 626/395-8111 X64297
Fax: 626/930-5394
www.cityofhope.org

Jonsson Comprehensive Cancer Center
University of California, Los Angeles
(Comprehensive Cancer Center)
Factor Building, Room 8-684
10833 LeConte Avenue
Los Angeles, CA 90095-1781
Tel: 310/825-5268
Fax: 310/206-5553
www.cancer.mednet.ucla.edu

UCSD Cancer Center
University of California at San Diego
(Comprehensive Cancer Center)
9500 Gilman Drive
LaJolla, CA 92093-0658
Tel: 858/822-1222
Fax: 858/822-0207
cancer.ucsd.edu

UCSF Cancer Center & Cancer Research Institute
University of California at
San Francisco
(Comprehensive Cancer Center)
2340 Sutter Street, Box 0128
San Francisco, CA 94115
Tel: 415/502-1710
Fax: 415/502-1712
cc.ucsf.edu

USC/Norris Comprehensive Cancer Center

University of Southern California
(Comprehensive Cancer Center)
1441 Eastlake Avenue, NOR 8302L
Los Angeles, CA 90033
Tel: 323/865-0816
Fax: 323/865-0102
ccnt.hsc.usc.edu

COLORADO
University of Colorado Cancer Center
University of Colorado Health
Science Center
(Comprehensive Cancer Center)
4200 East 9th Avenue, Box B188
Denver, CO 80262
Tel: 303/315-3007
Fax: 303/315-3304
uch.uchsc.edu/uccc/

CONNECTICUT
Yale Cancer Center
Yale University School of Medicine
(Comprehensive Cancer Center)
333 Cedar Street, Box 208028
New Haven, CT 06520
Tel: 203/785-4371
Fax: 203/785-4116
info.med.yale.edu/ycc/

DISTRICT OF COLUMBIA
Lombardi Cancer Research Center
Georgetown University Medical
Center
(Comprehensive Cancer Center)
3800 Reservoir Road, N.W.
Washington, DC 20007
Tel: 202/687-2110
Fax: 202/687-6402
lombardi.georgetown.edu

FLORIDA

H. Lee Moffitt Cancer Center &
Research Institute at the University of
South Florida
(Comprehensive Cancer Center)
12902 Magnolia Drive
Tampa, FL 33612-9497
Tel: 813/979-7265
Fax: 813/979-3919
daisy.moffitt.usf.edu

HAWAII

Cancer Research Center of Hawaii
University of Hawaii at Manoa
(Clinical Cancer Center)
1236 Lauhala Street
Honolulu, HI 96813
Tel: 808/586-3013
Fax: 808/586-3052
www.hawaii.edu/crch/

ILLINOIS

Robert H. Lurie Cancer Center
Northwestern University
(Comprehensive Cancer Center)
303 E. Chicago Avenue
Olson Pavilion 8250
Chicago, IL 60611
Tel: 312/908-5250
Fax: 312/908-1372
www.lurie.northwestern.edu/
index.html

University of Chicago Cancer
Research Center
(Comprehensive Cancer Center)
5841 S. Maryland Avenue, MC 1140
Chicago, IL 60637-1470

Tel: 773/702-6180
Fax: 773/702-9311
www-uccrc.bsd.uchicago.edu

INDIANA

Indiana University Cancer Center
(Clinical Cancer Center)
Indiana Cancer Pavilion
535 Barnhill Drive, Room 455
Indianapolis, IN 46202
Fax: 317/278-0074
iucc.iu.edu

Purdue University Cancer Center
(Cancer Center)
Hansen Life Sci. Research Bldg.
South University Street
West Lafayette, IN 47907-1524
Tel: 765/494-9129
Fax: 765/494-9193
www.cancer.purdue.edu

IOWA

Holden Comprehensive Cancer Center
University of Iowa
(Comprehensive Cancer Center)
5970 "Z" JPP
200 Hawkins Drive
Iowa City, IA 52242
Tel: 319/353-8620
Fax: 319/353-8988
www.uihealthcare.com/depts/
cancercenter/

MAINE

The Jackson Laboratory
(Cancer Center)
600 Main Street
Bar Harbor, ME 04609-0800

Tel: 207/288-6041
Fax: 207/288-6044
www.jax.org

MARYLAND

*The Sidney Kimmel Comprehensive
Cancer Center* at Johns Hopkins
(Comprehensive Cancer Center)
North Wolfe St., Room 157
Baltimore, MD 21287-8943
Tel: 410/955-8822
Fax: 410/955-6787
www.hopkinskimmelcancercenter.org

MASSACHUSETTS

Center for Cancer Research
Massachusetts Institute of
Technology
77 Massachusetts Avenue,
Room E17-110
Cambridge, MA 02139-4307
Tel: 617/253-8511
Fax: 617/253-0262
web.mit.edu/ccrhq/www/

Dana Farber/Harvard Cancer Center
Dana Farber Cancer Institute
44 Binney Street, Room 1628
Boston, MA 02115
Tel: 617/632-4266
Fax: 617/632-2161
www.dfci.harvard.edu/

MICHIGAN

*Barbara Ann Karmanos Cancer
Institute*
Wayne State University
Operating the Meyer L. Prentis
Comprehensive Cancer Center of
Metropolitan Detroit
(Comprehensive Cancer Center)

540 E. Canfield, Room 1241
Detroit, MI 48201
Tel: 313/577-1335
Fax: 313/577-8777
www.karmanos.org

Comprehensive Cancer Center
University of Michigan
(Comprehensive Cancer Center)
6302 CGC/0942
1500 E. Medical Center Drive
Ann Arbor, MI 48109-0942
Tel: 734/936-1831
Fax: 734/615-3947
www.cancer.med.umich.edu

MINNESOTA

Mayo Clinic Cancer Center
Mayo Foundation
(Comprehensive Cancer Center)
200 First Street, S.W.
Rochester, MN 55905
Tel: 507/284-3753
Fax: 507/284-9349
www.mayo.edu/cancercenter/center/

University of Minnesota Cancer Center
(Comprehensive Cancer Center)
MMC 806, 420 Delaware Street, S.E.
Minneapolis, MN 55455
Tel: 612/624-8484
Fax: 612/626-3069
www.cancer.umn.edu/

MISSOURI

Siteman Cancer Center
Washington University School of
Medicine
(Clinical Cancer Center)
600 S. Euclid Avenue, Box 8100

St. Louis, MO 63110-1093
Tel: 314/747-7222
Fax: 314/454-5300
medicine.wustl.edu/

NEBRASKA
University of Nebraska Medical Center
Eppley Cancer Center
(Clinical Cancer Center)
600 S. 42nd Street
Omaha, NE 68198-6805
Tel: 402/559-5238
Fax: 402/559-4652
www.unmc.edu/cancercenter/

NEW HAMPSHIRE
Norris Cotton Cancer Center
Dartmouth-Hitchcock Medical Center
(Comprehensive Cancer Center)
1 Medical Center Drive,
Hinman Box 7920
Lebanon, NH 03756-0001
Tel: 603/650-6300
Fax: 603/650-6333
www.dartmouth.edu/dms/nccc

NEW JERSEY
The Cancer Institute of New Jersey
Robert Wood Johnson Medical
School
(Clinical Cancer Center)
195 Little Albany Street, Room 2002B
New Brunswick, NJ 08901
Tel: 732/235-8064
Fax: 732/235-8094
cinj.umdng.edu/

NEW YORK
American Health Foundation
(Cancer Center)

300 E. 42nd Street
New York, NY 10017
Tel: 212/551-2500
Fax: 212/687-2339
www.ahf.org

Cancer Research Center
Albert Einstein College of Medicine
(Clinical Cancer Center)
Chanin Building, Room 209
1300 Morris Park Avenue
Bronx, NY 10461
Tel: 718/430-2302
Fax: 718/430-8550
www.aecom.yu.edu

Cold Spring Harbor Laboratory
(Cancer Center)
P.O. Box 100
Cold Spring Harbor, NY 11724
Tel: 516/367-8383
Fax: 516/367-8879
www.cshl.org/

Herbert Irving Comprehensive
Cancer Center
College of Physicians & Surgeons
Columbia University
(Comprehensive Cancer Center)
177 Fort Washington Avenue
6th Floor, Room 435
New York, NY 10032
Tel: 212/305-8602
Fax: 212/305-3035
www.ccc.columbia.edu

Kaplan Cancer Center
New York University Medical Center
(Comprehensive Cancer Center)
550 First Avenue
New York, NY 10016

Tel: 212/263-8950
Fax: 212/263-8210
www.nyucancerinstitute.org/
newlocation.html

Memorial Sloan Kettering
Cancer Center
(Comprehensive Cancer Center)
1275 York Avenue
New York, NY 10021
Tel: 212/639-6561
Fax: 212/717-3299
www.mskcc.org/mskcc/html/44.cfm

Roswell Park Cancer Institute
(Comprehensive Cancer Center)
Elm and Carlton Streets
Buffalo, NY 14263-0001
Tel: 716/845-5772
Fax: 716/845-8261
www.roswellpark.org/

NORTH CAROLINA
Comprehensive Cancer Center
Wake Forest University
Medical Center Boulevard
Winston-Salem, NC 27157-1082
Tel: 336/716-7971
Fax: 336/716-0293
www.bgsm.edu/cancer/

Duke Comprehensive Cancer Center
Duke University Medical Center
(Comprehensive Cancer Center)
Box 3843
Durham, NC 27710
Tel: 919/684-5613
Fax: 919/684-5653
www.cancer.duke.edu/

University of North Carolina at
Chapel Hill
(Comprehensive Cancer Center)
School of Medicine, CB-7295
102 West Drive
Chapel Hill, NC 27599-7295
Tel: 919/966-3036
Fax: 919/966-3015
cancer.med.unc.edu/

OHIO
Clara D. Bloomfield, M.D.
Director
Comprehensive Cancer Center
Arthur G. James Cancer Hospital &
Richard J. Solove Research Institute
Ohio State University
(Comprehensive Cancer Center)
A455 Staring Loving Hall
300 W. 10th Avenue
Columbus, OH 43210-1240
Tel: 614/293-7518
Fax: 614/293-7520

Ireland Cancer Center
Case Western Reserve &
University Hospitals of Cleveland
(Comprehensive Cancer Center)
11100 Euclid Avenue, Wearn 151
Cleveland, OH 44106-5065
Tel: 216/844-8562
Fax: 216/844-4975
www.irelandcancercenter.org/

OREGON
Oregon Cancer Center
Oregon Health Sciences University
(Clinical Cancer Center)
3181 S.W. Sam Jackson Park Road,
CR145

Portland, OR 97201-3098
Tel: 503/494-1617
Fax: 503/494-7086

PENNSYLVANIA
Fox Chase Cancer Center
(Comprehensive Cancer Center)
7701 Burholme Avenue
Philadelphia, PA 19111
Tel: 215/728-2781
Fax: 215/728-2571
www.fccc.edu/

Kimmel Cancer Center
Thomas Jefferson University
(Clinical Cancer Center)
233 S. 10th Street
BLSB, Room 1050
Philadelphia, PA 19107
Tel: 215/503-4645
Fax: 215/923-3528
www.kcc.tju.edu/

University of Pennsylvania Cancer
Center
(Comprehensive Cancer Center)
3400 Spruce Street
16th Floor Penn Tower
Philadelphia, PA 19104
Tel: 215/662-6065
Fax: 215/349-5325
pennhealth.com/health/hi_files/
cancer

University of Pittsburgh Cancer
Institute
(Comprehensive Cancer Center)
3550 Terrace Street, Suite 401
Pittsburgh, PA 15213

Tel: 412/648-2255
Fax: 412/648-2741
www.upci.upmc.edu/

The Wistar Institute
(Cancer Center)
3601 Spruce Street
Philadelphia, PA 19104
Tel: 215/898-3926
Fax: 215/573-2097
www.wistar.upenn.edu/

TENNESSEE
Vanderbilt-Ingram Cancer Center
(Comprehensive Cancer Center)
Medical Research Building II
Nashville, TN 37232
Tel: 615/936-1782
Fax: 615/926-1790
www.vanderbiltcancer.org/

TEXAS
San Antonio Cancer Institute
(Comprehensive Cancer Center)
7979 Wurzback Drive
Urscel Tower, 6th Floor
San Antonio, TX 78229
Tel: 210/616-5580
Fax: 210/692-9823
www.saci.org/

University of Texas
M. D. Anderson Cancer Center
(Comprehensive Cancer Center)
1515 Holcombe Boulevard, Box 91
Houston, TX 77030
Tel: 713/792-6000
Fax: 713/799-2210
www.mdanderson.org/

UTAH
Huntsman Cancer Institute
University of Utah
(Clinical Cancer Center)
2000 Circle of Hope
Salt Lake City, UT 84112
Tel: 801/585-3401
Fax: 801/585-6345
www.hci.utah.edu/

VERMONT
Vermont Cancer Center
University of Vermont
(Comprehensive Cancer Center)
149 Beaumont Avenue, HRSF326
Burlington, VT 05405
Tel: 802/656-4414
Fax: 802/656-8788
www.vermontcancer.org/

VIRGINIA
Cancer Center
*University of Virginia Health
Sciences Center*
(Clinical Cancer Center)
Jefferson Park Avenue, Room 4015
Charlottesville, VA 22908
Tel: 804/924-5022
Fax: 804/982-0918
www.med.virginia.edu/

Massey Cancer Center
Virginia Commonwealth University
(Clinical Cancer Center)
P.O. Box 980037
Richmond, VA 23298-0037
Tel: 804/828-0450
Fax: 804/828-8453
www.vcu.edu/mcc/

WASHINGTON
*Fred Hutchinson Cancer
Research Center*
(Comprehensive Cancer Center)
1100 Fairview Avenue, North
P.O. Box 19024, D1060
Seattle, WA 98104
Tel: 206/667-4305
Fax: 206/667-5258
www.fhcrc.org/

WISCONSIN
Comprehensive Cancer Center
University of Wisconsin
(Comprehensive Cancer Center)
600 Highland Avenue, Room K4/610
Madison, WI 53792
Tel: 608/263-8610
Fax: 608/263-8613

Breast Cancer Organizations

African American Breast
Cancer Alliance
612/825-3675

American Breast Cancer Foundation
877/539-2543
www.abcf.org

American Cancer Society
800/ACS-2345
www.cancer.org

American Society of Clinical Oncology
703/299-0150
www.asco.org

The Breast Cancer Care and
Research Fund
310/791-6295
www.breastcancercare.org

The Breast Cancer Fund
866/760-8233
415/346-8223
www.breastcancerfund.org

Cancer Research Institute
800/99-CANCER
www.cancerresearch.org

The Chemotherapy Foundation
212/213-9292

Corporate Angel Network, Inc.
914/328-1313
www.corpangelnetwork.org

Kids Konnected
800/899-2866
www.kidskonnected.org

Living beyond Breast Cancer
888/753-5222
www.lbbc.org

The Mautner Project for Lesbians
with Cancer
202/332-5536
www.mautnerproject.org

National Alliance of Breast Cancer
Organizations
888/80-NABCO
www.nabco.org

National Asian Women's Health
Organization
415/989-9747
www.nawho.org

National Breast Cancer Coalition
202/296-7477
www.natlbcc.org

National Cancer Institute
800/4-CANCER
www.nci.nih.gov

National Coalition for Cancer
Research
www.cancercoalition.org/main.html

National Coalition for Cancer
Survivorship
877/NCCS YES
www.cansearch.org

National Comprehensive Cancer
Network
888/909-NCCN
www.nccn.org

National Women's Health
Network
202/628-7814
202/347-1140
www.womenshealthnetwork.org

Native American Cancer Initiatives, Inc.
303/838-9359
members.aol.com/natamcan

Oncology Nursing Society
412/921-7373
www.ons.org

Patient Advocate Foundation
800/532-5274
www.patientadvocate.org

Susan G. Komen Breast Cancer
Foundation
800/462-9273
www.breastcancerinfo.com
www.komen.org

The Wellness Community
888/793-WELL
www.wellness-community.org

Y-Me National Breast Cancer
Organization
800/221-2141
800/986-9505 (Spanish)

Online Resources

Breast Cancer Information Core (BIC)
www.nhgri.nih.gov/Intramural
research/

California Breast Cancer Organizations
www.cabco.org

Cancer Information Network
www.cancernetwork.com

CancerLinks
510/649-8177
www.cancerlinks.org

CenterWatch, Inc. Clinical Trials
Listing Service
www.centerwatch.com

International Cancer Alliance
www.icare.org

Myriad Genetic Laboratories
www.myriad.com

National Cancer Institute CancerNet
www.cancernet.nci.nih.gov

National Coalition for Cancer
Survivorship
www.nccs.org

National Lymphedema Network
800/541-3259
www.lymphnet.org

OBGYN.net Latina
Latina.obgyn.net/español

Office of Minority Health Resource
Center
www.omhrc.gov

OncoLink—*Breast Cancer*
www.oncolink.upenn.edu/disease/
breast

Rational Therapeutics
www.rationaltherapeutics.com

Susan Love, M.D.
www.susanlovemd.com

*Vital Options TeleSupport Cancer
Network*
800/477-7666
www.vitaloptions.org

*Y-Me National Breast Cancer
Organization*
www.y-me.org

Books

Brinker, Nancy G., and Catherine McEvilly-Harris, *The Race Is Run One Step at a Time: Every Woman's Guide to Taking Charge of Breast Cancer.* New York: Simon & Schuster, 1990.

Canfield, J., M. V. Hansen, P. Aubery, and N. Mitchell, *Chicken Soup for the Surviving Soul.* Deerfield Beach, Fla.: Health Communications Inc., 1996.

Clegg, Holly, and Gerald Miletello, *Eating Well through Cancer.* Memphis, Tenn.: The Wimmer Companies, 2001.

Harpham, Wendy Schlossel, *After Cancer: A Guide to Your New Life.* New York: Norton, 1994.

Kaye, Ronnie, *Spinning Straw into Gold: Your Emotional Recovery from Breast Cancer.* New York: Simon & Schuster, 1991.

Link, John S., *The Breast Cancer Survival Manual: A Step-by-Step Guide for the Woman with Newly Diagnosed Breast Cancer.* New York: Owl Books, 1998.

Love, Susan M., with Karen Lindsay, *Dr. Susan Love's Breast Book*, 2nd ed. New York: Addison-Wesley, 1995.

Remen, Rachel Naomi, *Kitchen Table Wisdom.* New York: Riverhead Books, 1996.

———, *My Grandfather's Blessings: Stories of Strength, Refuge and Belonging.* New York: Riverhead Books, 2001.

Weihofen, Donna, with Christina Marino, *The Cancer Survival Cookbook.* New York: Wiley & Sons, 1997.

Weiss, Marisa C., and Ellen Weiss, *Living beyond Breast Cancer: A Survivor's Guide for When Treatment Ends and the Rest of Your Life Begins.* New York: Times Books, 1998.

Index

adjuvant systemic therapy, 25, 80, 81–82, 87, 145
adrenal glands, removal of, 88
adriamycin, 105–6
advocate for yourself, 8, 16, 17, 97, 104
age at diagnosis, 141
aggressive cancers, 21, 25, 62, 86, 107, 108, 146
  rating scale, 81, 85, 86
  in story, 22
alternative therapies, 60
American Cancer Society, 41, 130
anastrozole (Arimidex), 88
angiogenesis, 28, 95, 100, 101, 111
angiogenesis factors, 86
antiangiogenesis agents, 95
antibodies, 84, 86, 103, 108–9
antibody therapy, 25
antidepressants, 143
anti-VEGF, 111
apoptosis (cell death), 19, 21, 81, 86, 91, 95, 99, 101, 112
  loss of, 100
aromatase, 87
  aromtase inhibitors, 87, 88, 90, 111–12, 145
Astroglide, 143
atypical ductal hyperplasia (ADH), 32
atypical hyperplasia, 100

B14 study, 89
B20 study, 89
bacterial infection, 94
Baker, Jim, 14

basement membrane, 79, 100
Bazell, Robert, 110
beliefs, 126–27, 130, 131
bilateral mastectomy, 33, 115
  with reconstruction, 71, 72–74
  skin-sparing, 72–73
biopsy, 40, 44, 75–76, 119, 139
  pathology report from, 25
  see also needle biopsy
biopsy specimen, 139
blood vessel development, 83, 111
blood vessels, 25, 86
body
  changes in, 150, 151, 152, 153
  trust in, 119, 154
body image, 136, 151
bone marrow, 21, 84, 94
brain chemistry, 122–23
BRCA 1 and 2, 21, 32, 72, 98, 115, 117
breast
  location of cancer in, 139–40
  loss of, 141
  risk of cancer in uninvolved, 71
  saving, 68–77
breast cancer, 2, 8, 18, 28, 122
  beginning of, 18–21, 27, 79
  causes of, 118–19, 131–32
  demystifying, 17–29
  development of, 97–98
  estrogen dependent, 87, 88, 90
  as gift, 61
  mutated genes in, 98–101
  passing to offspring, 98
  prevention of second, 117

breast cancer (cont'd)
  sensitivity to chemotherapy, 91
  specialists in care of, 8–9
breast cancer characteristics, 62, 77
  for treatment planning, 26t
Breast Cancer Survival Manual, The
  (Link), 1, 5, 14, 21, 80
breast conservation, 9, 63, 77, 151
breast ducts, 27f
Breast Friends, 124
breast-conserving surgery, 68, 70, 71
  followed by radiation, 76
Breastlink.com, 5
Bruyere, Rosalyn L., 127–29

Calderwood, Lynette, 109–10
cancer(s)
  categorized by phenotypic nature, 19
  caused by mutations in DNA code,
    98
  changes life forever, 113
  removing, 138–39
  see also breast cancer; lobular cancers
cancer cells, 21
  circulating, 64
  dividing, 91
  escaped, 81, 83, 84, 96
  iatrogenic spread of, 85
  mutated, 93
  and external factors, 86–87
  pass altered DNA to progeny, 19
  penetrating basement membrane, 79
cancer centers, 40, 76, 77
cancer spread factors, 85–87
capitation, 11
care
  fragmentation of, 10–11
  follow-up, 113–17
  standard of, 2
  see also optimal care/treatment
Caswell, Dr., 22–23, 24
cell biology, 112
cell death
  see apoptosis (cell death)
cell division, 28, 80, 99–100, 101
  accelerated, 101–2
  interfering with, 91
cell types, 21, 81
cells, 19
  escaped, 25, 62
  malignant, 27–29

migration, 44
  mutations, 97–98
  well-differentiated, 28
change(s), 161
  from breast cancer, 136–37
  illness as agent of, 158
chemotherapy, 9, 13, 14, 44, 63, 83,
    105–6, 119, 122
  drugs, 23–24
  effects of, 136, 137, 153
  fatigue with, 125
  and ovarian failure, 146–48
  overutilized, 147
  preoperative, 23, 24, 65–66
  and reproductive capacity, 146
  routinely prescribed, 9–10
  sex and, 144–46, 154
  with spread to lymph system, 45
  in story, 79–80
  systemic therapy with, 25
  see also cytotoxic chemotherapy
choices, 3, 6, 76–77
clear margins, 28, 70, 137, 138, 140
clinical trials, 37, 60, 94, 95, 96, 112,
    126–27
clodronate, 95
control, 4–5, 6, 17, 124
  over body, 125
  of effects of breast cancer experience, 47
  loss of, 133, 159
cosmetic results, 63, 70, 139, 140
  good, 28, 68, 69
cost containment, 11, 15
crisis management, 119–20, 121, 122
"Culture of Healing, The," 130–31
cure, 59, 65, 83, 100, 161
  assessing probability of, 62–65
  issues of, 4
  potential for, 87
  after systemic relapse, 114
cure rate, 2, 8, 10, 59, 64, 90, 113, 149
cytotoxic chemotherapy, 89–90, 91–95
  classes of, 92–93
  and ovarian function, 147

death, 53, 61, 79, 159
  causes of, 116
death rate, 117
decision making
  complexity of, 79, 80
  factors in, 87

decisions, 6, 77, 119
  about care, 9
  empowerment for, 62
  informed, 67
  for systemic treatment, 81–85
  see also treatment decisions
depression, 4, 121, 122–23, 132
  in story, 60–61
diagnosis, 21, 28, 29, 30, 61, 118, 119,
    161
  choices about, 3
  effects on women, 78–79
  opportunity in, 6
  reaction to, 118, 119, 121–23, 124, 125
diagnostic imaging, 114
diet, 115–16, 124, 144
dirty margins, 139
DNA (deoxyribonucleic acid), 21, 97, 99
  abnormal fragment of, 108
  mutations in, 18, 19, 86, 98, 101
  protecting, 103
doctor/patient relationship, 5, 10, 58
doctors/physicians
  addressing whole person, 46, 47, 48
  capitated, 11
  coordination among, 4, 28
  disagreement among, 43
  empathy and sympathy, 57–58
  and faith/healing, 129
  in HMOs, 16
  are human, 5, 52–58
  knowledge of new treatments, 34,
    37–39
  mismanagement by, 7–8
  mistakes by, 15
  objectivity, 96
  and patient's reaction to diagnosis, 123
  side effects not addressed by, 137
  see also under specialty, e.g.,
    oncologist(s)
drug regimens, multiple, 93
drug resistance, 93
  genetic basis for, 83
drugs, 28, 86, 87, 105–6
  new, 38–39
ductal cancer in situ (DCIS), 64, 69, 70,
    85

education (patient), 2, 4, 5, 10, 75, 119
  demystifies breast cancer, 17
  about risks/benefits, 90

eggs, harvesting/storing, 148
emotional states, 4, 119, 121
empathy, 55, 56, 57
empowerment, 2, 17, 80, 131
endorphins, 124–25
Epidermal Growth Factor (EGF) genes,
    102
Epidermal Growth Factor Receptor
    (EGFR), 20t, 21
epithelial cells, 84
estrogen, 100
  as external factor, 86–87
  influence on breast cancer, 88, 89
  lack of, 142, 143, 153, 154
  and libido, 144
  replacement, 66
estrogen receptor-positive breast cancer,
    112, 117, 142, 148
estrogen receptors, 21, 27, 86, 88
exercise, 115–16, 124–25, 144, 146
existential crisis, 156–58

faith, 126–35
family, 122
family history, 33, 77, 114
Faslodex (fulvestrant), 112
fatigue, 153
fee for service system, 11, 16
femininity, 136
fertility, 4, 146–49
fibrocystic breasts, 75
fibrosis, 70
filgrastim (Newpogen), 94
5-hydroxytryptophan, 143
follow-up care, 113–17
Food and Drug Administration (FDA),
    95, 106, 107, 108
FSH (follicle-stimulating hormones), 148
Freud, Sigmund, 66

gain of function mutations, 101–3
Ganz, Patricia, 154
gatekeeper, 11
gene mutations, 80–81
  types of, 101–4
gene research, 86
gene therapy, 81, 99
Genentech, 108, 110, 111
genes
  altered, 86, 105
  mutated, 98–101

genetic cloning, 148
genetic mishaps, 18, 19, 100–101
   correcting, 111–12
genetic predisposition, 18
genetic risk, 97, 98
genetic testing, 72
genetics, 97–104, 105
   research based on, 112
genotypic analysis, 19
Getting Well Again (Simonton), 130, 131
glandular cell(s), 27, 98
Green, Elmer, 128
grief/grieving, 147, 151
growth factors, 28, 94, 108
guided imagery, 133
gynecologist, 155
gynecomastia, 143

hair loss, 136, 137, 144, 153
Halsted, William, 9
Halsted radical mastectomy, 9, 130
healing, 3, 4, 16, 47–48, 56
   from doctor's perspective, 53
   faith and, 126–35
   physical, 152
   styles for, 57
health care, 8, 11, 76
heart disease, 59, 116
Her-2 (Bazell), 110
Her-2/neu oncogene, 21, 86, 95, 102, 108
herbs, 146
Herceptin, 28, 86, 95, 99, 107–10, 111
hereditary risk, 32, 72
heterogeneity of breast cancer, 21, 25, 28,
   62, 100–1, 105, 148–49
HMOs, 4, 11, 42, 47
   in story, 11–16
hormonal changes, 4, 142–43, 144
hormonal therapy, 9, 25, 44, 63, 88–91
   with chemotherapy, 81
   classes of, 90–91
   protection against recurrence, 116
   see also hormone replacement therapy
      (HRT)
hormone receptor positive (ER+) cells,
   81
hormone receptor-negative cancers, 116,
   117
hormone receptor-positive cancers, 115,
   117, 147

hormone receptors, 27–28, 111
hormone replacement therapy (HRT),
   66–67, 115, 145
   discontinuing, 122, 142–43, 153
   new, 111–12
hot flashes, 66, 88, 115, 122, 142, 143,
   145–46
human drug testing, 106–7
   Herceptin, 108–10
human genome, 98–99
Human Genome Project, 99
Hunt, Valerie, 128
hydration, 93–94
hyperplasia, 99–100
hysterectomy, 143

Ibarra, Julio, 14
Ikiru (film), 156–58, 160
illness, 47, 56
   as agent of change, 158
   life-threatening, 156
imagery
   focused, 130, 133
imaging, 16, 25, 114, 139
imaging techniques, new, 45
implant(s), 70, 73–74
implant enhancement surgery, 141
in situ cancer, 21, 100
   see also ductal cancer in situ (DCIS)
incision(s), 69f, 73, 139, 140
   placement of, 70, 138
inflammatory breast cancer, 23, 64
information, 21, 77, 87, 96
   sources, 80
innovations, 34–36
insurance, 3, 4, 44, 151
intercourse, painful, 66, 142
interval cancers, 25
interventions, 79, 96
intratumor heterogeneity, 81

Jonsson Comprehensive Cancer Center,
   110
jungle floor model of drug development,
   105–6

Kegel exercises, 143, 154
Ki-67 status, 21
Kurosawa, Akira, 157
Kushner, Rose, 76

learned helplessness, 131
LeShan, Lawrence, 132
letrozole (Femara), 88
LHRH (luteinizing hormone-releasing
    hormone) agonist/antagonist drugs,
    88, 90, 148
libido, 115, 144, 146
life
    after breast cancer, 149
    with breast cancer, 136–49
    limited, 158–60, 162
    living, 159–60, 162
    as miracle, 135
    mystery of, 162
    precious and short, 61
    reviewing, 156
life situation
    and loss of breast, 141
life-stress scale, 132
ligands, 101
lobular cancers, 69–71, 114, 115
    in story, 71
lobular cells, 27f
lobular neoplasia, 117
local control, 4, 9, 44, 76, 151
    with breast-conserving surgery, 68,
        69
    options for, 74
    surgery for, 28
local recurrence rate, 10
loss, 151
    addressing, 152
loss of function mutations, 101, 102, 103
lubricants, 143, 154
lumpectomy, 44, 68, 119, 151
Lupron, 88
lymph node dissection, 45
    in story, 22
lymph nodes, 62, 64, 65, 84
    cancer cells in, 85
    cancer spread to, in story, 22, 23, 24,
        25
lymphoma, 14, 15
lympho-vascular index, 21

mammograms, 33, 114, 119, 138
    reviewing, 40, 139
    see also screening mammography
managed care, 15–16, 23, 46–47
Maslow, Abraham, 33

mastectomy, 9, 23, 25, 44, 64–65, 68–69,
    70, 76, 119, 141, 151
    decision for, 77
    incisions, 137–38
    as only option, 75
    prophylactic, 72, 74
    see also bilateral mastectomy; radical
        mastectomy
medical care delivery industry, 4
medical oncologist(s), 32, 52, 63, 114,
    119
medical oncology, 9
medical system, 7
medications, new, 95, 96
    see also drugs
medicine, 162
    forces influencing, 31
    perspectives on, 129–30
Menninger Clinic, Center for Applied
    Psychophysiology, 128
menopausal symptoms, 122, 142, 146,
    153
menopause, 88
    premature, 122, 145, 146
metastatic disease, 83, 96, 145
metastatization, 79, 100
micro-array analysis, 101
micrometastatic disease, 81–83, 82f,
    94–95
mind, 118–25
miracles, 133–35
misdiagnosis, 7, 14
Modified Bloom Richardson scale
    (MBR), 81
modified radical mastectomy, 74, 75
molds, 105, 106
mood disturbances, 88, 142–43
mortality, 156
    see also death
MRI, 33, 114
multidisciplinary team/review, 31–32,
    33–37
mutation(s), 18, 86
    see also gene mutations
Myriad Genetic Laboratories, 72

nadir count, 94
National Cancer Institute (NCI), 40, 41
National Surgical Adjuvant Breast and
    Bowel Project, 89

needle biopsy, 28, 63, 75–76
    advantages of, 138
    information from, 25
    spreading cells, 83, 85
    in story, 22
neo-adjuvant chemotherapy, 25, 63–64
neoplasia, 115
nipple-areolar complex, 140

oncogenes, 101, 103, 108
oncologist(s), 3, 9–10, 13–14, 32, 37, 43,
        52, 117, 147, 155
    consulting, 39–40
    use of chemotherapy, 89
oncology, 57, 58
one-stage mastectomy, 75, 76
optimal care/treatment, 2–3, 4, 5, 25, 31,
        33–34, 61, 161
    achieving, 8–9
    advocating for, 16
    defined, 7
    difficulty receiving, 8
    doctors in, 28
    inhibitors to, 34
    participation with, 131
    women do not receive, 53
options, 10, 77
    information regarding, 71
    in surgery, 68
    see also treatment options
Osler, William, 54
osteoporosis, 115
ovarian ablation, 88–89
ovarian failure, 146–47
ovarian suppression, 89, 90, 136, 142, 147
ovaries
    protecting, 147–48
    removed, 88
overexpression, 108
overtreatment, 2, 6, 10, 18
ovulation, suppressing, 148

P53 gene, 21, 86, 103
partner(s), 122, 144
    effects of your breast cancer on,
        150–52
    and loss of breast, 141
pathologist(s), 9, 28, 32, 63, 138
pathology, 16, 40, 62
pathology report(s), 25

patient
    causing disease, 131–32
    as decision maker, 10, 76
    doctors learning from, 55
    and life-enhancing/diminishing
        experience of breast cancer, 47, 48
    in new research, 112
Paxil, 143
peer mentoring programs, 77, 124
Perelman, Ronald, 110
pharmaceutical industry, 4, 5, 37, 111
    and doctors, 38–39
phenotypic characteristics, 19–21, 20t
physical appearance, 141, 152
physicians
    see doctors/physicians
phyto estrogens, 146
plastic surgeon/surgery, 32, 70, 1141
postmenopausal women, 112
    and HRT, 142, 145
    and libido, 144
post-traumatic stress disorder, 121
precancerous phases, 99, 100–101
pregnancy, 147
pretreatment planning conference,
        32–37
prevention trials, 116–17
primary care physician (PCP), 11, 12, 13,
        137
progesterone, 27, 145–46
    replacement, 66, 88
progesterone receptors, 21, 27, 88
prognosis, 19, 107
prognostic factors, 20t
progress, 3, 5, 74–75, 155
protein receptors, 101, 103
proteins, 18, 28, 99, 101, 102
    abnormal, 62, 107–8, 111
    blood-vessel stimulating, 111
    new, 95–96, 100
Prozac, 143
psychotherapist/psychotherapy, 3, 9, 121,
        155

quality of life, 4, 62, 96, 114–15, 121,
        122, 145, 157
    adjustments in, 142
    assessing, 65–67
    after diagnosis, 59
    after treatment, 153–54

quality-of-life issues, 137, 146
quantity of life, 96

radiation, 119, 140
    fatigue with, 125
    with surgery, 70, 76
radiation oncologists, 9, 10, 32, 52, 130
radiation therapy, 10, 68, 69
    protection against recurrence, 116
    follow-up, 139
radical mastectomy, 9, 75, 130
    in story, 22
radiologist(s), 9, 32, 52, 114
    bracketing the cancer, 138–39
Raloxifene, 115, 116, 117
Reagan, Nancy, 77
reconstruction, 70, 71, 77, 151
    immediate, 64
    immediate, with bilateral mastectomy,
        72–74
    optimal, 138
recurrence, 4, 10
    fear of, 114
    protective factors against, 116–17
relapse, 62, 82, 83, 85
    in pregnancy, 147
    preventing systemic, 116
    risk of, 79, 84
relapse rate, 64, 65
Replens, 143
reproduction, 146–49
reproductive endocrinology, 148
research, 31, 76, 87
    current trends in, 105, 107
    human genome, 99
    in naturally occurring compounds, 116
    new, 112
resilience, 119, 120
resources, 77, 169–79
Revlon Breast Center, 110
risk assessment, 59–60, 62, 77, 78–96
risk factors, 114
risk of second cancer, 114, 115–16
risk pool, 11
risks/benefits, 4
    of chemotherapy, 10, 94
    education regarding, 90
    of HRT, 66–67, 115
    of systemic treatment, 80
running energy, 128, 129

St. John's wort, 143
scars/scarring, 2, 8, 68–69, 75, 136,
        137–40, 152
    anxiety about, 152
    peri-areolar, 140
    in story, 74
Schain, Wendy, 76
scientific method, 129
screening mammography, 10, 24–25
    in story, 22
second opinion, 8, 14, 15, 16, 28, 48, 79,
        151
    getting, 39–42
    getting results of, 42–44
    guidelines for, 40–41
    importance of, 31–33
    sources for, 40
Seligman, Martin, 131
sentinel lymph node staging, 37–38
sentinel node, 37, 38, 85
    locating, 45
sentinel node technique, 79
SERMs (selective estrogen receptor
        modulators), 88, 90, 115, 116–17
serotonin depletion, 122–23, 142
sex
    and chemotherapy, 144–46
sexual desire, decrease in, 142, 153
sexuality, 4, 136–37
    renewing, 150–55
side effects, 106, 117
    adjuvant systemic therapy, 87
    aromatase inhibitors, 145
    chemotherapy, 93, 95, 137, 147
    cytotoxic chemotherapy, 89
    hormonal changes, 142–43
    hormonal therapy, 88
    recovery from, 8
    tamoxifen, 145–46
silastic ring, 143, 154
Simonton, O. Carl, 130, 131, 133
skin-sparing procedure, 73, 73f, 140
Slamon, Dennis, 107–8, 109, 110
soy, 146
specialists/specialization, 9, 44, 46, 147,
        148
    working together, 29, 32
specialty blinders, 33–34
spiritual healer(s), 127–28, 129
SSRI antidepressants, 143

standard of care, 2
STAR trial, 117
statistical analysis, 62, 87, 89, 96
statistical probability, 72
  treatment based on, 81
stem cells, 91
Stephens, Loren, 55–56
stories, 5
  addressing whole person, 48–51
  author's mother/sister, 1, 3, 11–15, 16,
    22–25, 57
  bilateral mastectomy with immediate
    reconstruction, 72–74
  chemotherapy, 79–80
  faith and healing, 127–28
  finding meaning in cancer, 120–21
  Herceptin, 109–10
  lobular cancer, 71
  miracles, 133–34
  second opinions, 32–33
  survival, 60–61
stress
  and cancer, 132–33
stromal cells, 147
stromal tissue, 100
support, 2, 122
support programs, 123–24
surgeon(s), 3, 9, 28, 32, 43, 52
  create scars, 137–38
  general, 63, 75–76
  radiologist and, 138–39
  and sentinel lymph node technique, 38
surgery
  options in, 68–77
  radiation with, 70, 76
  reconstructive, 70
  and scarring, 137–40
  second, third, 28, 138
  spreading cells, 83
  tissue removal in, 69–70
  when and where to operate, 139–40
surgical preventive strategies, 117
surveillance, 33, 113–14, 117
survival, 8, 59–67, 140
  five-year, 65, 114
  phenotypic characteristics and, 19
  twenty-year, 85
survivors, 155, 158
sympathy, 55, 56, 57
systemic relapse, preventing, 116
systemic risk, assessing, 63

systemic spread, 9, 10, 82
  risk of, 62, 79, 85
systemic therapy/treatment, 4, 9, 25, 44,
    63–64, 146
  classes of, 87, 88–96
  decision for, 81–85
  hormonal manipulation, 147
  prior to surgery, 28–29, 140
  risks/benefits, 80

Tabar, Laszlo, 85
tamoxifen, 88, 89, 90
  and libido, 144–45
  and reproductive capacity, 146
  tests, 116–17
Tartikoff, Lilly, 110
taxanes, 23
technology, new, 4, 34–36t, 103
testosterone, 88, 145–46
  and libido, 144
tests/testing, 106–7, 111
  in follow-up care, 114
  Herceptin, 108–10
  needed, 62, 81, 83, 95, 96
  new, 84
  tamoxifen, 116–17
  see also clinical trials
therapies
  alternative, 60
  new, 111
  see also systemic therapy/treatment;
    treatment
toremifene, 88
touch, 152–53
toxic effects/toxicity, 4, 81, 93, 106, 107,
    144
transformation, 157, 158, 159, 160
  opportunities for, 122
trauma, meaning in, 120–21
treatment, 2, 8, 17, 19, 29
  addressing genetic errors, 97
  based on nature of breast cancer, 8, 18
  changing, 45
  choices about, 3, 77
  future, 103–4
  getting most current, 37–39
  inappropriate, 6–7
  in managed care, 15
  new, 34–37
  proceeding with, 44–45
  questions in, 96

requirements of, 28
right, 30–31
sequence of, 44
and sexuality, 153–54, 155
unnecessary, 83
see also optimal care/treatment
treatment agents, new, 105–17
treatment decisions, 6, 119
  body image in, 151
treatment information, 5
treatment modalities, combining, 81
treatment options, 59–60
  for whole woman, 74–75
treatment plan/planning, 25, 29, 31,
    44–45, 60, 119
  characteristics for, 26t
  disagreement about, 43
  hormone receptor status in, 27–28
  initial, 39, 42
treatment process, 3–4
treatment team, 47–48
trust, 4–5, 52
tumor behavior, prediction of, 81–83, 84
tumor size, 21
tumor volume, 85

UCLA
  Institutional Review Board, 108
  Laboratory of Applied Kinesiology, 128
ultrasound, 33, 40, 114

uniqueness, 4, 21, 29, 62, 80, 121–22
University of Southern California, 129
urinary incontinence, 143
urinary tract infection, 66, 142
uterine cancer, 117

vagina, 88, 142, 153
vaginal atrophy, 154
vaginal dryness, 115, 136, 143, 146
variables, 21
vascular endothelial growth factor
    (VEGF), 21, 111
visualization, 130, 133
vitamin supplements, 115

weight gain, 136, 137
Weil, Andrew, 128
white blood count, 94
whole person, treating, 46–51, 52, 75,
    161
wide local excision, 68
women
  with breast cancer, 1–2, 7–8
  health issues, 76

Y-Me Support Group, 42
yoga, 146

Zoladex, 88
Zoloft, 143

About the Author

JOHN LINK, M.D., is the medical director of one of the leading breast cancer treatment centers in Southern California. He has been honored by the American Cancer Society for his commitment to the treatment and cure for breast cancer. He is the author of *The Breast Cancer Survival Manual*.